Meeting the Challenges of Oral and Head and Neck Cancer

A GUIDE FOR SURVIVORS AND CAREGIVERS

Second Edition

Meeting the Challenges of Oral and Head and Neck Cancer

A GUIDE FOR SURVIVORS AND CAREGIVERS

Second Edition

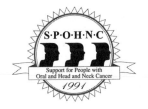

Edited by
Nancy E. Leupold, MA
James J. Sciubba, DMD, PhD

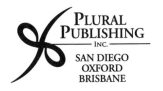

PLURAL
PUBLISHING
INC.
SAN DIEGO
OXFORD
BRISBANE

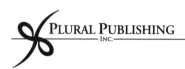

PLURAL PUBLISHING
INC.

5521 Ruffin Road
San Diego, CA 92123

e-mail: info@pluralpublishing.com
Web site: http://www.pluralpublishing.com

49 Bath Street
Abingdon, Oxfordshire OX14 1EA
United Kingdom

Copyright © by Plural Publishing, Inc. 2008

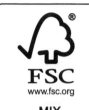

FSC
www.fsc.org
MIX
Paper from
responsible sources
FSC® C011935

Typeset in 11/13 Garamond by Flanagan's Publishing Services.
Printed in the United States of America by McNaughton & Gunn.
Cover Design by Réne Rodriguez, Rhino Graphics LLC

Library of Congress Cataloging-in-Publication Data

Meeting the challenges of oral and head and neck cancer : a survivor's guide
/ [edited by] Nancy E. Leupold & James Sciubba. — 2nd ed.
   p. cm.
  Includes bibliographical references and index.
  ISBN-13: 978-1-59756-454-0 (alk. paper)
  ISBN-10: 1-59756-454-0 (alk. paper)
  1. Head—Cancer—Patients—Rehabilitation. 2. Neck—Cancer—Patients—
Rehabilitation. I. Leupold, Nancy E. II. Sciubba, James J.
  RC280.H4M4 2011
  616.99'491—dc23

                        2011026999

CONTENTS

v

FOREWORD

We welcome the second edition of *Meeting the Challenges of Oral and Head and Neck Cancer: A Guide for Survivors and Caregivers*. Much important information on the subject has become available in the decade since the first edition. This volume has been expanded, updated, and polished and thus constitutes an even more comprehensive resource of valuable scientific, psychological, sociological, therapeutic, financial, and practical information for the patient afflicted with head and neck cancer and his or her family. The original text extensively has been rewritten and made more comprehensive.

Five new chapters provide important and exciting new information. First among them is the description of the emerging role of human papillomavirus (HPV) in the genesis of oropharyngeal cancer with important therapeutic and prognostic implications. The next describes the introduction of robotic surgery in the therapeutic attack on oropharyngeal and laryngeal cancer and the advantages and limitations thereof. The third new chapter more extensively addresses the important and complex matter of pain management in the head and neck cancer patient. The next addition deals with the challenges of quality of life, a matter of special importance to the head and neck cancer patient as the disease and its treatment often profoundly impact the patient's personal image and vital functions including communication, eating, and swallowing. The last addition addresses the challenges of the psychological effects and sequellae of head and neck cancer. All patients suffer psychological consequences of the disease and its treatment, but many will require additional dedicated and appropriate treatment for the anxiety, depression, and concerns about coping ability.

With the addition of this new and expanded information to the updated original chapters, this guide provides even more valuable information, practical advice, and recommendations in addition to an extensive list of references, resources, support groups, and Web sites. These are valuable for the patients and their families, but also will provide helpful and valuable information not generally available for otolaryngological nurses, physicians' assistants, and other health personnel providing care for these patients.

The basic principles of complete care of the head and neck cancer patient have not changed and include, but are not limited to, the following:

A. The vital importance of the doctor/patient relationship characterized by good and continuing two-way communication;
B. The importance of good education about, and understanding of, the disease and its treatment by the patient and family;
C. The importance of the "captain" of the ship, the physical leader of the entire treatment team, and of his or her continuing availability to the patient and family;
D. The primacy of quality of life considerations as part of all educational and therapeutic decision-making.

Appreciation of these principles and others too numerous to mention will soften the impact of the cancer and facilitate the care of, as well as the caring for, the patient afflicted with head and neck cancer.

> Elliot W. Strong, MD, FACS
> Emeritus, Memorial Hospital for Cancer and Allied
>   Disease
> Emeritus, Memorial Sloan Kettering Cancer Center
> Former Attending Surgeon and Chief, Head and
>   Neck Service
> Former Professor of Surgery at Cornell University
>   Medical College

PREFACE

Head and neck cancers comprise a variety of malignant tumors that may occur in the head and neck region, namely the oral cavity, the pharynx (throat), the cervical esophagus, the paranasal sinuses and nasal cavity, the larynx, and the thyroid and the salivary glands. Lesions of the facial skin, scalp, and neck and the cervical lymph nodes also may be classified as head and neck cancers.

Although the prevalence of oral and head and neck cancer in the United States is only about 3 to 4% of all cancers diagnosed, the importance of these diseases is heightened by the fact that functional problems and esthetic differences are commonly associated with this type of cancer and its treatment. Indeed, coping with oral and head and neck cancer can be extremely difficult. Not only is a person dealing with a diagnosis that can be life-threatening, but he or she must also deal with possible alterations in facial appearance, speech, and the senses of smell and taste, swallowing, and vision. These alterations, in turn, may lead to considerable threats to one's self-image, confidence, identity, and emotional balance. No body part is so exposed to the world as a person's face, head, and neck. Other scars and deformities of the body may be covered, but it is difficult to hide disfigurements and treatment-associated dysfunctions of the oral cavity and head and neck.

As a result of the ongoing changes in the treatment of oral and head and neck cancer and the use of the Internet to obtain information, patients and their families are becoming increasingly more active in researching and identifying their options for care. The capability of patients more actively to participate in

their own care has increased the need for education and awareness of the various and often overwhelming information that is
available through the Internet. This level of patient empowerment
has begun to change the doctor-patient relationship with the
patient and family being more involved than ever in treatment
decisions and understanding the levels of risk and anticipated
benefits of proposed treatment.

Since the founding of Support for People with Oral and Head
and Neck Cancer (SPOHNC) in 1991, we have had the opportunity to speak with thousands of survivors who have undergone
various treatments for their cancers. Most discover that there are
only limited and reliable resources available to them concerning head and neck cancer. This, in turn, has led patients and
their families to contact SPOHNC for help in finding answers to
specific questions related to their individual cancer journeys in
thoughtful and patient-directed ways.

*Meeting the Challenges of Oral and Head and Neck Can-
cer: A Survivor's Guide,* published in 2008, offered the patient,
caregiver, family, and friends the opportunity to learn about a
difficult cancer and its associated treatment options as well as
some of the psychosocial aspects of living with the disease and
its aftermath. Information concerning dental care, skin care,
communication and swallowing difficulties, nutrition, insurance
issues, and clinical trials also was included in this book. This
second edition, *Meeting the Challenges of Oral and Head and
Neck Cancer: A Guide for Survivors and Caregivers* provides
updates on many of the chapters and includes an additional five
new chapters on subjects that are of importance to this population. As in the first edition, there is an extensive chapter which
includes tables of products, therapies, and survivor input providing information and supportive care to head and neck cancer
survivors facing the challenges of side effects or lingering effects
of treatment.

*Meeting the Challenges of Oral and Head and Neck Cancer:
A Guide for Survivors and Caregivers* is written in user-friendly,
patient-directed language about oral and head and neck cancer.

With all that this book encompasses, it is a "must-have" additional reference for survivors, caregivers, family, and friends as well as health care professionals involved in the management of oral and head and neck cancer patients.

Nancy E. Leupold, M.A.
Survivor, President and Founder
SPOHNC

James J. Sciubba, D.M.D., Ph.D
Vice President and Chairman, Medical Advisory Board
SPOHNC

ACKNOWLEDGMENTS

Meeting the Challenges of Oral and Head and Neck Cancer: A Survivor's Guide first was introduced to the public in 2008. Now, three years later, we are pleased to present a second edition of the book entitled *Meeting the Challenges of Oral and Head and Neck Cancer: A Guide for Survivors and Caregivers.* This edition contains five new chapters as well as updates of the original chapters.

SPOHNC is most appreciative of the many authors who have contributed to this new book. Their contributions of chapters and sections of *Meeting the Challenges of Oral and Head and Neck Cancer: A Guide for Survivors and Caregivers* make this new publication a comprehensive resource for oral and head and neck cancer survivors, their caregivers, and health care professionals.

Many survivors, family members, and health care professionals offered suggestions and input to the content, resources, and tables in this book. We greatly appreciate the contributions of John Acton, Belinda Andrews, Trisha Appelhans, Sandra Ashley, Sandy Bates, Joseph R. Bauer, Charlie Bauer, Janis Beard, Michael Birnbaum, Lawrie Bloom, Patricia M. Boldt, Mary Grace Bontempo, Stephen Bortz, Boston Chapter, Richard Boucher, Addie Brown, Sheryl Bunton, Rita Burfitt, Emily and Dennis Carroll, Kathleen A. Castillo, John M. Chambers, Kathy Chambers, Barry Cooper, Lillian Corbett, Gene Covington, Joan Cummings, David Curbello, Dallas Chapter, Allison Dekker, RN, Hank V. Deneski, Bette L. Denlinger, Sal and Jean Diana, Jane Dien, John P. Dowling, Gail Fass, Evelyn Fowler, Gerry Frankel, Peach Gazda, Vince Gilhool, Karyl L. Gill, Carol Glavin, Mike Golub, Lynn Gormley, John Groves, Elizabeth Hadas, Marilyn Haines,

Gabriel Hamilton, Jean Harrison, Michael Henault, Jerry Hepburn, Dave Hepburn, Harry G. Hives, Pam Hoff, Henry V. Holdridge, Carol Humphries, Jack and Temple Igleburger, Indianapolis South Chapter, Neal Isaacs, Kansas City Chapter, Dianne Kiyomoto-Kuey, RD, Robert R. Klauber, Brent Koehler, Lee Laino, Jeffrey Langdale, Sherry Laniado, Leonard Lanyo, Pat Laumann, Janice Leak, Linda Legendre, Danny Lindburg, Ann Linkh, Los Angeles-UCLA Chapter, Robin Luo, Gail B. Mackiernan, Araik Margarian, Carolyn Martocchia, Joe Meditz, Larry Menkoff, Martha Miller, Thomas E. Momeyer, Dwayne and Barbara Moore, Micki Naimoli, Lisa and Tuan Nguyen, NJ-Philadelphia Chapter, Bill Parisi, Monica Pfister, Sherry Pinkof, Pat and Felix Quinn, Phil E. and Naomi Reimer, Sharon A. Renkes, Sanford Riesenfeld, Jerome P. Rothstein, DDS, MHA, Jerry Runyon, Ernst Schneck, E. J. Scott, Joann Scott, Bob Simpson, Sister Mary Ryan, SP, Sandra L. Smith, Dan Stack, Dennis Staropoli, Alice Steiner, Nancy Symonds, RDH, Valerie Doreen Targia, Sharon Tupa, Ronnie Trentham, George Tyson, Chuck Van Alen, Janet Wallstadt, Madelyn Walsh, Mike Yelinek, Mark H. Weiss, Bill and Ann Wesp, Sheila West, Allen Wilson, Mary Ellyn Witt, RN, Jan Wundsam, Tom Yohe, and the many others who through the years have shared their stories and provided support and encouragement to others.

And for reviewing and helping to provide information for the "tables" and "resources," we gratefully acknowledge the work of SPOHNC's staff: Mary Ann Caputo, Executive Director, Chris Leonardis, Outreach Administrator, and Lisa Caracciola, Administrative Assistant.

For support and encouragement of this new book, we also wish to thank the Board of Directors and the Medical Advisory Board of SPOHNC.

Meeting the Challenges of Oral and Head and Neck Cancer: A Survivor's Guide began as an idea for bringing practical information to oral and head and neck cancer survivors in a reader-friendly format. In this new edition, *Meeting the Challenges of Oral and Head and Neck Cancer: A Guide for Survivors and Caregivers,* we are pleased to expand the content of this book to address the issues and treatments of 2011.

CONTRIBUTORS

Shrujal Baxi, MD, MPH
Physician
Memorial Sloan-Kettering Cancer
  Center
New York, NY
Chapter 6

Julie Blair, MA, CCC-SLP
Clinical Instructor
Evelyn Trammell Institute for
  Voice and Swallowing
Adjunct Faculty
College of Health Professions
Medical University of South
  Carolina
Charleston, South Carolina
Chapter 12

David M. Brizel, MD
Professor of Radiation Oncology
Associate Professor of
  Otolaryngology Head and
  Neck Surgery
Duke Comprehensive Cancer
  Center
Duke University Medical Center
Durham, North Carolina
Chapter 5

**Sandy Cavell, PGDipSci,
PGDipHealthPsych, MA
(Hons), MSc (Hons)**
Health Psychology
Otolaryngology

Manukau Superclinic
Manukau Central, New Zealand
Chapter 11

Patty Delaney[†]
Former Director
Cancer Liaison Programs
Food and Drug Association
Chapter 15B

Kendrea L. Focht, CScD
Doctoral Student
Medical University of
  South Carolina
Charleston, South Carolina
Chapter 12

Gail Funk, RN, OCN
Clinical Nurse IV
Department of Radiation
  Oncology
Duke University Hospital System
Durham, North Carolina
Chapter 5

Matthew G. Fury, MD, PhD
Assistant Attending Physician
Memorial Sloan-Kettering Cancer
  Center
New York, New York
Chapter 6

Linda Gilliard, MS, RD, CNSD
Clinical Dietitian

[†]Deceased

Radiation Oncology Clinic
Duke University Medical Center
Durham, North Carolina
Chapter 5

Dorothy Gold, MSW, LCSW-C, OSW-C
Senior Oncology Social Worker
Milton J. Dance, Jr. Head and
   Neck Cancer
Greater Baltimore Medical Center
Baltimore, Maryland
Chapter 10

Patrick K. Ha, MD, FACS
Assistant Professor
John Hopkins Department of
   Otolaryngology
John Hopkins Head and Neck
   Surgery
Greater Baltimore Medical Center
Baltimore, Maryland
Chapter 2

Malinda Heuring
Director of Education
National Foundation for
   Ectodermal Dysplasias (NFED)
Mascoutah, Illinois
Chapter 14B

Pat Jolley, RN, BS
Chief of Patient Services
Patient Advocate Foundation
Hampton, Virginia
Chapter 14A

Mario E. Lacouture, MD
Assistant Professor
Director, Cancer Skin Care Program
Department of Dermatology
Robert H Lurie Comprehensive
   Cancer Center

Northwestern University
Chicago, Illinois
Chapter 8

Nancy E. Leupold, MA
Survivor, President and Founder
Support for People with Oral
   and Head and Neck Cancer,
   (SPOHNC)
Madison, New Jersey
Chapters 15A and 16

Su Hsien Lim, MD
Head and Neck Medical
   Oncology Fellow
Memorial Sloan-Kettering Cancer
   Center
New York, New York
Chapter 6

Elaine C. Martinez, LPN
Patient Advocate Foundation
San Antonio, Texas
Chapter 14

Bonnie Martin-Harris, PhD, CCC-SLP, BRS-S
Director, MUSC Evelyn Trammell
   Institute for Voice and
   Swallowing
Associate Professor,
   Otolaryngology-Head and
   Neck Surgery
Medical University of South
   Carolina
Charleston, South Carolina
Chapter 12

Deborah J. Miller, PhD, MPH, RN
Cancer Liaison Program
Food and Drug Administration
Office of Special Health Issues

Silver Spring, Maryland
Chapter 15B

Erin Moaratty
Chief of External Communications
Patient Advocate Foundation
Hampton, Virginia
Chapter 14A

Randall P. Morton, MB, BS, MSc, FRACS
Professor of Otolaryngology-
    Head and Neck Surgery
University of Auckland
Consultant Otolaryngologist-
    Head and Neck Surgeon
Counties-Manukau District
    Health Board
Manukau Central, New Zealand
Chapter 11

Barbara A. Murphy, MD
Associate Professor of Medicine
Director, Head and Neck
    Research Team
Director, Pain and Symptom
    Management Program
Vanderbilt-Ingram Cancer Center
Nashville, Tennessee
Chapter 9

Eugene N. Myers, MD, FACS, FRCS Edin. (Hon)
Distinguished Professor and
    Emeritus Chair
Department of Otolaryngology
University of Pittsburgh School
    of Medicine and Medical
    Center
Pittsburgh, Pennsylvania
Chapter 3

David Myssiorek, MD, FACS
Professor of Otolaryngology
New York University School of
    Medicine
New York, New York
Chapter 1

Tammy Neice, RN
Senior Clinical Case Manager
Patient Advocate Foundation
Hampton, Virginia
Chapter 14A

Bert W. O'Malley, Jr, MD
Professor and Chairman
Otorhinolaryngology-Head and
    Neck Surgery
University of Pennsylvania
    Health Care System
Philadelphia, Pennsylvania
Chapter 4

Beth Patterson
President, Mission Delivery
Chief of Patient Services
Patient Advocate Foundation
Hampton, Virginia
Chapter 14A

David G. Pfister, MD
Chief, Head and Neck Medical
    Oncology Service
Co-leader, Head and Neck Cancer
    Disease Management Team
Memorial Sloan-Kettering Cancer
    Center
Professor of Medicine
Weill Medical College of Cornell
    University
New York, New York
Chapter 6

Mary Kaye Richter
Executive Director and Founder
National Foundation for
   Ectodermal Dysplasias (NFED)
Mascoutah, Illinois
Chapter 14B

Mary Ann Downey Rubio
Senior PA-C
Department of Radiation
   Oncology
Duke University Medical Center
Durham, North Carolina
Chapter 5

James J. Sciubba, DMD, PhD
The Milton J. Dance Head &
   Neck Cancer Center
The Greater Baltimore Medical
   Center
Baltimore, Maryland
Professor, Ret. The Johns
   Hopkins Medical School
Department of Otolaryngology,
   Head and Neck Surgery
Chapter 7

Brandey Terruso, RN, CSO, LDN
Clinical Dietitian
Duke University Hospital
Radiation Oncology Clinic
Durham, NC
Chapter 5

**Jennifer Thompson, RD, LD,
   CNSD**
Senior Clinical Dietitian
Department of Oncology and
   Blood and Marrow Transplant
Baylor University Medical Center
Dallas, Texas
Chapter 13

Tanya Walker, RN, BSN
Senior Clinical Case Manager
Patient Advocate Foundation
Newport News, Virginia
Chapter 14A

Gregory S. Weinstein, MD
Professor and Vice Chairman
Director, Division of Head and
   Neck Surgery
Abraham Cancer Center
University of Pennsylvania
   Health Care System
Philadelphia, Pennsylvania
Chapter 4

David S. Yoo, MD, PhD
Medical Instructor
Department of Radiation
   Oncology
Duke University Medical Center
Durham, North Carolina
Chapter 5

1

INTRODUCTION TO THE CHALLENGES OF ORAL AND HEAD AND NECK CANCER

David Myssiorek, MD, FACS

Head and neck cancer (HNC) encompasses a group of tumors that arise from the structures of the upper aerodigestive tract. Classically, these structures are involved with swallowing, speaking, and breathing (mouth, throat, nose, sinuses, larynx, and upper esophagus); salivary glands (parotid gland, submandibular gland, sublingual gland, and minor salivary glands); thyroid gland and parathyroid glands; and the ear, and skin of the head and neck. Additionally, the lymph nodes of the neck are always considered when dealing with cancers of these organs. Diverse tumors, both benign and malignant, can arise from these structures. Many different salivary gland tumors and thyroid tumors are found yearly, but the most common cancer of the head and neck in adults is squamous cell carcinoma. Squamous cell carcinoma arises from the cells that line the upper aerodigestive tract, sinuses, and skin. This resource book addresses the treatments and their aftereffects for people with head and neck cancer.

Anatomy

The subsites of the upper aerodigestive tract include the mouth, nose, sinuses, pharynx, larynx, and neck. The oral cavity starts at the exposed margins of the upper and lower lips called the vermilion border which shares a sharp border with the adjacent skin. Because of a rich vascular supply to the lip and a thin covering, the vermilion appears redder than skin. The mucous membrane covering the cheeks and lips running from the upper gum to the lower gum lines is known as the buccal mucosa. A triangular area extending medially (inward) to the region between the buccal mucosa and the space between the upper and lower gum is called the retromolar trigone. The oral cavity ends at the junction of the hard and soft palates, with the oropharynx beginning at this point and extending into the throat.

The tongue is divided into thirds. The front two-thirds of the tongue is considered a structure of the oral cavity and is responsible for speech, articulation, and taste and also helps to move food to the teeth for chewing and backward for swallowing. The undersurface of the tongue (ventral tongue) blends into the floor of the mouth. The floor of the mouth is located between the dental-bearing tissues of the lower jaw and bears the ducts of both submandibular glands (Diagram 1–1). The alveolar ridge is the structure that contains the teeth and gums.

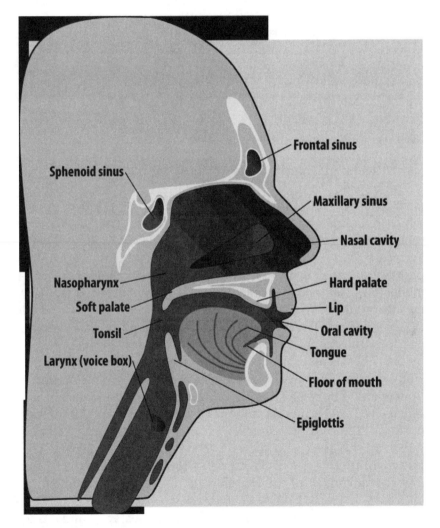

Diagram 1–1. Basic anatomy of the head and neck. Courtesy of the American Society for Therapeutic Radiology and Oncology (ASTRO).

There is a lower (mandibular) alveolus and upper (maxillary) alveolus. The hard palate marks the posterior extent of the oral cavity. To a degree, oral cavity structures develop from embryologic structures arising from the cranial nerve associated with mastication (chewing).

The pharynx is divided into three regions: the nasopharynx, the oropharynx, and the hypopharynx. The nasopharynx begins at the choanae, the portals at the back of the nasal cavity that transmit air, and is continuous with the posterior wall of the oropharynx. The lateral walls contain the eustachian tube openings that extend to the middle ear. A cleft between this opening and the posterior wall known as the fossa of Rosenmüller is a frequent site of cancer. The anterior or front wall of the nasopharynx is the back of the soft palate.

Descending from the nasopharynx is the oropharynx. The lateral or side walls contain the tonsils. The anterior border is partially made up of a ring of tissue known as Waldeyer's ring, which contains abundant tonsillar-type tissue. The base of the tongue (posterior third) and the tonsils are part of Waldeyer's ring, an area rich in lymphoid tissue. The soft palate is the remaining part of the anterior border. The inferior border includes attachments to the larynx by various folds and ligaments. An imaginary line through the hyoid bone demarcates the inferior border of the oropharynx. The hypopharynx is roughly funnel shaped and is continuous with the oropharynx above and the esophagus below. The recesses lateral to the larynx are called pyriform sinuses, which are pyramidal in shape with the apexes pointed downward. The pyriform sinuses have a medial and lateral wall. The medial wall abuts the superior half of the larynx. The upper border of the pyriform sinus is the pharyngoepiglottic fold and inferiorly the apex is at the cricoid cartilage of the larynx. The postcricoid area is the back end of the lower portion of the larynx that contains most of the muscles that move the vocal folds.

The larynx forms at the end of the trachea and "buds" into the pharynx during embryogenesis. The larynx is made of bone, cartilage, and muscle. It is divided into a superior or upper half, which is mostly sensory (allowing perception of food/liquid before it enters the windpipe), but there is little motor function. The epiglottis acts as a keel to divert food and liquid to the sides away from the laryngeal opening. The inferior or lower half contains the motor parts of the larynx—the vocal folds. The space between them is the glottis. The vocal folds form a complex valve that allows us to hold our breath and block matter from entering the lungs. When these folds are damaged or paralyzed, aspiration can occur. Secondarily, the vocal folds are responsible for voice. The vocal folds are attached to the thyroid cartilage anteriorly and to the arytenoid cartilages posteriorly. The arytenoid cartilages can move side to side and front to back and thus are capable of moving the vocal folds in complex ways, creating the human larynx's range of sounds. All of the muscles attached to the arytenoids are innervated by the recurrent laryngeal nerve, which is a major branch of the vagus nerve.

Incidence

The incidence of HNC has stabilized. In 2010, there were 36,540 new cases of cancer of the oral cavity and pharynx, approximately one-third in the tongue, one-third in the mouth, and one-third in the oropharynx and pharynx (Jemal et al., 2010). Another 12,700 cases were predicted in the larynx and 44,670 cases in the thyroid. Comparatively, during this same year, 222,520 lung cancers, 217,730 prostate cancers, and 209,060 breast cancers were estimated. Oral cavity and pharyngeal cancers account for 3% of all cancers in men and less than 1% in women. From 1991 to 2003, the death rate for these tumors decreased from 2.03 per 100,000 women to 1.47 per 100,000 women, representing an overall change of 27% in women. Similarly, men have experienced a drop from 5.61 per 100,000 to 4.06 per 100,000, representing an overall change of 27%. In men, death from laryngeal cancer has also decreased. There has been an improvement in the 5-year survival rate for the oral cavity (all stages included) from 53% in 1975 to 60% in 2002 (Jemal et al., 2010).

Etiology

Risk factors for the development of head and neck cancer include tobacco use (smoking, chewing, and snuff forms of smokeless tobacco) and reverse smoking (Decker & Goldstein, 1982), where smoking with the lighted end of the cigarette is placed inside the mouth; alcohol consumption (Strome et al., 2002); betel nut/paan chewing; and sun exposure of the lips and skin. Other suspected etiologies include human papillomavirus (D'Souza et al., 2007; Licitra et al., 2006; Snijders et al., 1992), reflux disease (Locke, Talley, & Fett, 1999; Qadeer, Colabianchi, Strome, & Vaezi, 2006), and a familial predisposition (Copper et al., 1995). Some evidence exists that some laryngeal cancers may be related to occupational risks (Brown et al., 1988; Flanders & Rothman, 1982).

Squamous cell cancer represents more than 95% of all cancers of the upper aerodigestive tract. It is commonly associated with smoking and/or alcohol abuse. It is estimated that a person who smokes has 15 to 20 times the risk for developing head and neck cancer whereas alcohol abuse carries 2 to 3 times the risk for HNC. P53 is a tumor-suppressor gene whose mutation is associated with the development of upper aerodigestive tract cancer. These genetic mutations increase with smoking and drinking. Ninety-five percent of HNC is found in smokers. In Southeast Asia the practice of placing areca nut, spices, and tobacco along with lime paste into a betel leaf wrapping (paan) and chewing this has been linked to a large number of oral cavity cancers. In Mumbai approximately 50% of head and neck cancers are buccal cancers related to this practice. Chewing paan increases the risk of developing HNC by 2.8 times, and this number rises dramatically when chewing paan is combined with smoking, as often is the case in India.

Human papillomavirus (HPV) types 16 and 18 have been found in laryngeal verrucous cancers and tongue base and tonsil cancers. In a study from the Mayo Clinic (Strome et al., 2002), 46% of tonsil cancers examined had HPV DNA identified in the cancer cells. Only 6% of normal tonsils had HPV DNA copies.

Most recently, studies have been published that have confirmed this relationship in which the specific etiology of oropharyngeal squamous carcinoma was strongly linked with oropharyngeal HPV infection with or without the known associated risk factors of tobacco use and alcohol consumption (D'Souza et al., 2007).

Nasopharyngeal cancer is the most common cancer in China and is associated with a rise in the titer of anti-Epstein-Barr viral capsid antigens antibodies. The risk of people in Kwang Tung Province developing nasopharyngeal cancer is 25 times that of a Caucasian population. When people migrate from Kwang Tung, the increased risk of cancer persists but is decreased.

Some authors believe that some laryngeal cancers may be linked to laryngopharyngeal reflux (LPR) (Locke et al., 1999; Qadeer et al., 2006). The evidence supporting a direct cause and effect of LPR and laryngeal cancer is lacking at this time (Qadeer et al., 2006). Many earlier studies were poorly controlled. LPR has been found in approximately 40% of the U.S. population. Both smoking and alcohol consumption increase the likelihood of reflux (Locke et al., 1999). It is extremely difficult to isolate LPR as a cause of cancer.

Sun exposure is a known cause of both melanoma and other skin cancers, including basal cell and squamous cell cancers. The lips are particularly prone to squamous cell cancer from sun exposure.

Squamous Cell Carcinoma

Several types of cancers affect the lining of the upper aerodigestive tract. Besides squamous cell cancer, minor salivary gland cancers (adenocarcinomas), and metastases from other cancers can involve the head and neck. Squamous cell cancer is graded by the level of cellular differentiation. Well-differentiated cancers resemble the original cell from which they arose. Squamous cells line our mouths and throats, our sinuses, and all of our skin. It is a "wear and tear" lining and is waterproof. It produces keratin, which can readily be found in cuticles, nails, and hands and feet. Cancer of this cell type occurs when its DNA is altered and the cell proliferates in an independent or ungoverned fashion. Well-differentiated cancers tend to behave better than poorly differentiated cancers, in that they grow at a reduced rate compared to those that are less differentiated. The less differentiated a cell is, the less like the cell of origin it appears and the more invasive it becomes. The differentiation of the cancerous cell does not affect staging and is not often a predictor of outcome.

Variants of squamous cell carcinoma reflect special differentiation such as spindle cell or glandular differentiation. One variant, papillary carcinoma, behaves differently at the micro- and macroscopic level. Verrucous carcinoma closely resembles a wart, is slow growing, and rarely metastasizes but is locally destructive and frequently mistaken for more benign tumors. Generally, however, squamous cell cancer and its variants behave similarly and are treated similarly.

Squamous cell cancer starts as a clone of cells that reside within the epithelium or lining and proliferates within this layer initially. When limited to this epithelium, the entity is known as carcinoma in situ or CIS. If these cells invade through the basement membrane (a layer of collagen and glycoproteins that supports the epithelium and separates it from the underlying connective tissue), it is considered to be invasive and gains the potential to spread to regional lymph nodes in the neck and beyond.

Two terms require explanation. *Leukoplakia* is any white patch on a mucous membrane that doesn't wipe off. It usually indicates a state of damage or tissue alteration. It does not necessarily mean cancer as irritation by devices such as dentures and local trauma can result in leukoplakia. *Erythroplakia* is a velvety red lesion found on mucous membranes. This is usually more sinister than leukoplakia and requires investigation by biopsy.

A major concept in modern diagnosis and treatment is that of field cancerization (Slaughter, Southwick, & Smejkal, 1953). Simply put, whatever allowed one cell to differentiate or become cancerous (environment, irritants, radiation, genetics) can readily induce the same effect in other cells. This is why some patients develop multiple cancers within the upper aerodigestive tract. It is estimated that 20% of head and neck cancer patients will develop a second cancer in either the mouth, larynx, esophagus or lung. During the evaluation of a patient with head and neck cancer, physicians may order imaging studies and perform *pan-endoscopy* (a combination of laryngoscopy, esophagoscopy, and bronchoscopy) to seek out these second primary cancers.

Treatment Modalities

Treatment of head and neck cancer must take several factors into consideration. The age and health of the patient frequently determine how aggressive treatment can be. Some patients with liver disease from alcohol abuse often cannot tolerate certain chemotherapy regimens. The older patient with significant heart disease and other forms of medical compromise may not be able to tolerate a very lengthy cancer operation and reconstruction. Patients who already have had radiation therapy usually cannot get additional radiation therapy to the same area. Patients with Fanconi's anemia frequently have adverse reactions to radiation therapy, making it difficult to deliver such treatment safely (Bagby & Alter, 2006). The size of the lesion helps determine the clinical stage of the disease, which in turn will affect most treatment plans and overall prognosis. Patients with metastases to the neck require more therapy, usually a combination of treatment modalities, Distant metastases (lung, liver, bone, and brain) usually portend a poor outcome, with major surgical procedures not undertaken in this situation with unusual exceptions.

Treatment is determined by a multidisciplinary team in most locations in the United States. Tumor boards serve in an advisory fashion and consist of otolaryngologists, head and neck surgeons, plastic and reconstructive surgeons, radiation oncologists, medical oncologists, oral surgeons, pathologists, prosthodontists, nurses, speech-language pathologists, social workers, residents, and students. Early lesions (stages I and II) can usually be treated effectively by either radiation therapy or surgery. Later stage lesions (stages III and IV) usually require at least two treatment modalities, that is, radiation therapy and surgery or radiation therapy and chemotherapy. Many methods are used to determine the extent of disease prior to treatment planning. CT scan, MRIs, nuclear medical scans, endoscopy and biopsy, physical examination, and analysis of patient symptoms all enter into the evaluation of the cancer and, hence, the treatment plan.

Head and neck cancers and their treatment differ from other human cancers in several ways. Because the majority of head and neck cancers are tobacco and/or alcohol related, it is clear that most of these cancers are preventable. The structures of the head and neck are necessary for breathing, speaking, eating, hearing, seeing, smelling, and tasting. We contact our environment mainly through the head and neck. Cancers of this region and their treatment may result in deficits of any of these structures and their corresponding function. The person with oral and head and neck cancer requires greater rehabilitation, emotional support, and quality of life improvement than patients with most other cancers. In recent years, strides have been made to emphasize the important roles of prevention, early detection and treatment, and reconstruction of head and neck cancer defects. These efforts have resulted in decreasing numbers of many forms of head and neck cancer, improved quality of life, and improved survival rates.

References

Bagby, G. C., & Alter, B. P. (2006). Fanconi anemia. *Seminars in Hematology, 43,* 147–156.

Brown, L. M., Mason, T. J., Pickle, L. W., Stewart, P. A., Buffler, P. A., Burau, K., . . . Fraumeni, J. F., Jr. (1988). Occupational risk factors for laryngeal cancer on the Texas Gulf Coast. *Cancer Research, 48,* 1960–1964.

Copper, M. P., Jovanovic, A., Nauta, J. J., Braakhuis, B. J., de Vries, N., van der Waal, I., . . . Snow, G. B. (1995). Role of genetic factors in the etiology of squamous cell carcinoma of the head and neck. *Archives of Otolaryngology-Head and Neck Surgery, 121,* 157–160.

Decker, J., & Goldstein, J. C. (1982). Risk factors in head and neck cancer. *New England Journal of Medicine, 306,* 1151–1155.

D'Souza, G., Kreimer, A. R.,Viscidi, M., Pawlita, M., Fahkry, C., Koch, W. M., . . . Gillison, M. L. (2007). Case-control study of human papillomavirus and oropharyngeal cancer. *New England Journal of Medicine, 356,* 1944–1956.

Flanders, W. D., & Rothman, K. J. (1982). Occupational risk for laryngeal cancer. *American Journal of Public Health, 72,* 369–372.

Jemal, A., Siegel, R, & Ward, E. (2010). Cancer statistics, 2010. *CA: A Cancer Journal for Clinicians,* 60, 277–300.

Licitra, L., Perrone, F., Bossi, P., Suardi, S., Mariani, L.,Artusi, R., . . . Pilotti, S. (2006). High-risk human papillomavirus affects prognosis in patients with surgically treated oropharyngeal squamous cell carcinoma. *Journal of Clinical Oncology, 24,* 5630–5636.

Locke, G. R., III, Talley, N. J., & Fett, S. L. (1999). Risk factors associated with symptoms of gastroesophageal reflux. *American Journal of Medicine, 106,* 642–649.

Qadeer, M. A., Colabianchi, N., Strome, M.,& Vaezi, M. F. (2006). Gastroesophageal   reflux and laryngeal cancer: Causation or association? A critical review. *American Journal of Otolaryngology, 27,* 119–128.

Slaughter, D. P., Southwick, H. W., & Smejkal, W. (1953). "Field cancerization" in oral stratified squamous epithelium. *Cancer, 6,* 963–968.

Snijders, P. J., Cromme, F. V., van den Brule, A. J., Schrijnemakers, H. F., Snow, G. B., Meijer, C. J., . . . Walboomers, J. M. (1992). Prevalence and expression of human papillomavirus in tonsillar carcinomas, indicating a possible viral etiology. *International Journal of Cancer, 51,* 845–850.

Strome, S. E., Savva, A., Brissett, A. E., Gostout, B. S., Lewis, J., Clayton, A. C., . . . Kasperbauer, J. L. (2002). Squamous cell carcinoma of the tonsils: A molecular   analysis of HPV associations. *Clinical Cancer Research, 8,* 1093–1100.

Additional Reading

Anderson, S. R., & Sinacori, J. T. (2007). Plummer-Vinson syndrome heralded by postcricoid carcinoma. *American Journal of Otolaryngology, 28,* 22–24.

Gillison, M. L., & Shah, K. V. (2001). Human papillomavirus-associated head and neck squamous cell carcinoma: Mounting evidence for an etiologic role for human papillomavirus in a subset of head and neck cancers. *Current Opinion in Oncology, 13*, 183–188.

Hammarstedt, L., Lindquist, D., Dahlstrand, H., Romanitan, M., Dahlgren, L. O., Joneberg, J., . . . Munck-Wikland, E. (2006). Human papillomavirus as a risk factor for the increase in incidence of tonsillar cancer. *International Journal of Cancer, 119*, 2620–2623.

Hobbs, C. G., Sterne, J. A., Bailey, M., Heyderman, R. S., Birchall, M. A., & Thomas, S. J. (2006). Human papillomavirus and head and neck cancer: A systematic review and meta-analysis. *Clinical Otolaryngology, 31*, 259–266.

Vachin, F., Hans, S., Atlan, D., Brasnu, D., Menard, M., & Laccourreye, O. (2004). Long-term results of exclusive chemotherapy for glottic squamous cell carcinoma complete clinical responders after induction chemotherapy. *Annales d'Otolaryngologie et de Chirurgie Cervico-Faciale, 121*, 140–147.

2

MEETING THE CHALLENGES OF THE HUMAN PAPILLOMAVIRUS AND OROPHARYNGEAL CARCINOMA

Patrick K. Ha, MD, FACS

Human papillomaviruses (HPV) are a broad set of over 100 different infectious and transmissible viruses that exist in humans with various implications. These diverse subtypes can cause everything from common warts to cancer. Although recent research has pinpointed HPV type 16 to be most commonly implicated with oropharyngeal cancer, there is much that remains to be learned. In this brief chapter, we survey much of what is known about this disease process and what the future may bring. However, it should be understood that this is a rapidly evolving field, with new discoveries emerging every month. Although we have not drastically changed the way we approach patients with HPV-related head and neck cancer as of yet, there are different implications that require more in-depth conversations between you and the team taking care of you.

HPV in Cervical Cancer

HPV was first discovered as a cancer-related agent in cervical cancer, which is one of the most common malignancies throughout the world. It is felt that high-risk HPV subtypes cause up to 99% of cervical cancers (Stanley, 2010). Other cancers of the anogenital tract have also been linked with HPV, including vulvar, vaginal, penile, and anal cancers. Mucosal trauma to the epithelial lining is believed to provide the entrance portal for the virus preferentially infects these cells (Veldhuijzen, Snijders, Reiss, Meijer, & van de Wijgert, 2010). The infected cells can thus produce infectious viruses that are shed from the surface lining and evade the underlying immune system.

The lifetime risk of cervical HPV infection is 80%, and the majority of these infections of high-risk subtypes can be cleared within 2 years. As one might surmise, given the locations where these viruses tend to reside, HPV is a sexually transmitted disease. Because of varying sexual practices, the prevalence of cervical HPV is highest in the younger age groups and then declines with age. In men, the prevalence of genital HPV is difficult to determine due to differential sampling methods and selection bias. There is clear evidence that HPV may be transmitted to and from both partners with a higher degree or efficiency of transmission from the female to the male. Although males may serve as both the reservoir and vector for HPV transmission, the likelihood of penile cancer, for example, is quite rare. Infection through nonsexual contact is also up for debate; however, for now, it is widely believed to be predominantly sexually transmitted (Veldhuijzen et al., 2010).

HPV infection is thought to occur within the basal and more superficial layers of the mucosal lining, which are generally shielded by the multiple layers of differentiated or fully mature cells. However, when these overlying cells become disrupted through local trauma, the basal cells are exposed and vulnerable to infection. The basal cells are typically where the HPV reside. As these basal cells divide and head toward the surface lining, the virus has the opportunity to continue the replication process and lead toward further infection. The infection itself is a slow process, further allowing evasion of the virus from the host immune system (Horvath, Boulet, Renoux, Delvenne, & Bogers, 2010).

The development of cancer through HPV transformation is a slow process and may take years or even decades to form. In cervical cancer, the cells generally progress from a series of premalignant changes before turning into malignancy. This gradual process allows for possible detection, through the use of Papanicolaou (Pap) smears whereby cervical cell smears can be examined on a routine screening basis, with early intervention then undertaken as necessary. This has had a significant impact on decreasing the incidence of cervical cancer by as much as 70% (Veldhuijzen et al., 2010).

Mechanism of Cancer Formation

It was the research in the field of cervical cancer that led to the discovery of the molecular mechanism of HPV's role in causing cancer to form. When the virus infects a cell, it often sits outside the nucleus in a near-silent (episomal) state, until the cells migrate toward the surface, when it can churn out multiple copies of itself, which can then be shed and infect other cells. It may also integrate into the DNA of that cell, and when it does so, much of the viral genome, or DNA, is lost, except for two proteins, called the E6 and E7 proteins, which remain. It is these proteins that can lead to cancer formation. Interestingly, as integration of the virus occurs, the majority of the HPV genome is lost, and the actual cancer cells lose their ability to infect other cells, whereas the premalignant lesions retain their ability to cause infections (Conway & Meyers, 2009).

The E6 protein disrupts the p53 gene, which is the quintessential tumor-suppressor gene. This gene is responsible for the manufacture of p53 protein, the main regulator of apoptosis, or programmed cell death. Cells in the body generally are predetermined to have a certain life span, or when damaged, are supposed to die so that they do not cause further injury. However, when the p53 gene is disrupted and its protein is no longer available or is defective, these cells do not go through the planned cell death pathway and thus can live in perpetuity, potentially leading to cancer.

The second important HPV-related product, the E7 protein, disrupts the Rb gene, which is one of the DNA checkpoint genes that normally lead to cell death. Rb is a regulating protein that determines whether a cell's DNA has been damaged enough to warrant arrest, meaning that it would cause the cell to die. When this pathway is disrupted, the cell lacks this proofreading ability and can live on and grow in an unchecked fashion, thus leading to greater cancer susceptibility, as the damaged DNA can lead to mutations.

Of course, this is a very simplified account of how HPV infection can lead to cancer. However, regardless of the location of the HPV-associated cancer, it appears that the E6 and E7 genes from the virus and their products play a similar role in all of these and thus are the common basis for cancer development. The susceptibility for carcinogenic DNA mutations and other alterations is created by the E6 and E7 genes and increases the chances for cancer development to occur, although this may take years to develop.

HPV in Oropharyngeal Carcinoma

Understanding the association between high-risk HPV and oropharyngeal cancer (tonsil and tongue base) began in the late 1990s (Gillison, 2004). Several studies demonstrated similar findings of the presence of HPV DNA in oropharyngeal tumors with varying incidence. Most studies in the United States now find about 50 to 60% of cancers of the oropharynx to contain HPV DNA (Hennessey, Westra, & Califano, 2009). Now that this has been established, laboratory studies also indicate that similar molecular mechanisms are present in these cancers, namely, the presence of the E6 and E7 proteins and concomitant p53 and Rb inactivation. As in cervical cancer where HPV has a predilection toward involving the transformation zone, it appears to have a strong tendency to affect only lingual (tongue base) and palatine tonsillar tissues. For example, HPV has not consistently been identified in the oral part of the tongue, or that portion of the tongue that sits in the mouth at rest or in laryngeal cancers, despite the fact that screening studies have identified HPV infection in healthy individuals in about 4% of the time, with the high risk HPV-16 type involved in about 1% of presumably transient oral infections (Kreimer et al., 2010). Thus, one might conclude that, although HPV is often present, exposure to it rarely leads to cancer formation.

Although head and neck cancers are most often thought to affect patients who use tobacco and alcohol, the trend toward increased HPV-related oropharyngeal cancers in the United States has led to a shift in this patient demographic or subgroup. Patients with HPV-positive cancers tend to be younger, non-smokers, and nondrinkers. As HPV infection is thought to be sexually transmitted, there are associations with a younger age at first sexual contact, number of sexual partners, and oral/genital or oral/anal contact. It thus is postulated that viral transmission through sexual contact is likely and that the lymphoid tissue in the oropharynx, including the tongue base, is the final resting site of the virus. Therefore, the detection of oral HPV infection is likely to precede the development of oropharyngeal cancer, and work is being done to further refine the nature of exposure, the frequency, and the risk involved (Fakhry & Gillison, 2006).

Because HPV is most notably located in the anogenital tract, associations of HPV-associated cervical disease in the patient or significant other have been made, which was one of the first reasons why this was studied. Indeed, there is some evidence that women with cervical cancer are at somewhat elevated risk for the development of a second primary oropharyngeal cancer (Hennessey, Westra, & Califano, 2009). However, although this risk is elevated, oropharyngeal cancer remains relatively uncommon. Unfortunately, these findings do raise the possibility of transmission to others depending on sexual practice, but these associations remain limited and poorly studied.

Clinical Impact

There have been numerous retrospective reviews as well as prospective trial data indicating that individuals with HPV-associated head and neck cancer are generally: nonsmokers, nondrinkers, younger, and healthier than the typical head and neck cancer patient where tobacco and alcohol play a significant causative role. In addition, and importantly, HPV has been shown to be independently, positively associated with a better disease-free survival in large randomized trials in patients treated with primary chemoradiation. HPV-positive patients have up to a 60 to 80% reduction in risk of death from their head and neck cancer than HPV-negative patients (Chung & Gillison, 2009). It isn't clear why such benefit is conferred, but it likely is due to the difference in the mechanism of cancer development that renders these tumors to be more sensitive to chemotherapy and/or radiation therapy. In addition, patients are less likely to develop second smoking-related cancers such as other upper aerodigestive tract malignancies.

Although there is nearly universal acceptance of the evidence for a better prognosis and treatment response in nonsmoking patients with HPV-positive cancer, the question is what to do with this information. At the very least, when studies report their findings, it is now commonplace to indicate how many patients are HPV-positive as an indicator of what the treatment group was like, just as one might report the age or stage of the patients treated. However, as patients with HPV-related disease tend to fare better and are younger to begin with, more discussions have focused on the side effects of rigorous treatments and how these people will manage their long-term morbidity with potential swallowing dysfunction, xerostomia, taste disturbance, and so forth. As such, future chemoradiation trials have been proposed to reduce the dose of radiation when treating HPV-positive patients, although it should be cautioned that this would only be on a trial basis and not yet considered the standard of care. The introduction of less invasive transoral surgical techniques also may be more integrated into the treatment pathway. As patients who are HPV-negative tend to do worse, perhaps these patients would be better off with up-front surgery and postoperative chemoradiation as needed.

Thus far, we have been obtaining HPV status for information and prognostic purposes only, but not necessarily changing our patient management. One last point is that although HPV positivity appears to be associated with better survival, HPV positivity does not confer equal benefit in patients who smoke. Rather, there is evidence of a more "simple" or less virulent form of cancer that previously has not been associated with significant tobacco usage.

HPV Vaccines

Because of the knowledge that HPV is a highly transmissible disease, there has been the development of HPV preventive vaccines, which are designed to prevent or limit HPV infection. These vaccines have been created because of the high incidence of cervical cancer in the United States and throughout the world. They typically cover the high-risk HPV subtypes and are quite effective in providing host protection from the virus. Not only do they protect the individual, but also there is one less carrier who has the ability to spread the virus to others such that, over time, it may be possible to drastically reduce the incidence of HPV worldwide. Although preventive vaccines ultimately may have a substantial effect in cervical cancer, it is not known whether these vaccines will have any effect in reducing HPV-associated head and neck cancer. As it is the same HPV subtype responsible for susceptibility to malignancy in all of these cases, it is likely that, as vaccination becomes more widespread, we will see a concomitant reduction in the incidence of oropharyngeal head and neck cancer (Gillison, Chaturvedi, & Lowy, 2008).

The vaccines currently available are preventive vaccines, meaning that they should be used in individuals early on to provide protection from HPV infection. Another exciting area of vaccine research is the development of compounds that selectively may target HPV and cause cell killing in a specific manner. If able to isolate killing of just HPV-infected tumor cells, one could greatly enhance the effect while reducing side effects of those innocent, noninfected cells that are not involved. Thus, many researchers are looking into the creation of such products with the hope of someday being able to impact the treatment of these cancers. Again, as these patients typically are younger and healthier, these targeted compounds have the potential to offer a better long-term quality of life.

Patient Counseling

The diagnosis of head and neck cancer is overwhelming, but in discussing what is known about HPV and oropharyngeal cancer, there is still much that is unknown. In the cervical cancer literature, it is common that patients with HPV infection often feel anger, depression, isolation, fear of rejection, shame, and guilt. They also have fears about sexual contact and/or transmission to their partner (Anhang, Goodman, & Goldie, 2004). The same issues are likely to be true in patients with head and neck cancer, but unfortunately, even less is known about the details of many of these questions.

I believe that it is important to make patients aware of what we do know and to pre-emptively address some of the issues. It is important to realize that the HPV infection likely preceded the cancer by years, if not decades, as this sometimes can lead to questions of infidelity. It may be transmissible, although we have a poor understanding of the life cycle of the HPV in the oral cavity. It is important for women who have or are partnered with male patients with HPV-related or pharyngeal cancer to continue with routine Pap smears and cervical exams. As it is still rare that couples should both develop oropharyngeal cancer, I do not necessarily discourage intimate contact. I do encourage individuals to consider the HPV vaccine for their children, with the understanding that it may not necessarily impact the risk for head and neck cancer development, but it will have an effect on the incidence of cervical cancer.

Clearly, many unanswered questions still exist, as we have only begun to recognize the potential nuances of treating HPV-related head and neck cancers. We still do not fully understand the significance of oral HPV infection and how that necessarily leads to the development of oropharyngeal cancer. Is there a premalignant phase that typically is seen in cervical cancer common to oropharyngeal cancer that might allow for earlier detection? Is there a significant transmissibility risk from patients with HPV-associated disease to their loved ones? Will the current HPV vaccines have a substantial impact on head and neck cancer along with cervical cancer? It is of the utmost importance that the patient and family be given reliable information about HPV and its impact on clinical outcomes and social interactions.

Conclusion

In summary, there have been great strides in the descriptive nature of HPV-associated head and neck cancers. These appear to be specific to the oropharynx (tonsil and tongue base regions), and affect a different patient demographic than in the past. Patients tend to fare better, opening the door to potential changes in the manner in which they are treated, but this has not yet been proven in large clinical trials. Preventive HPV vaccination may alter future incidence, and we hope that meaningful therapeutic vaccines will be forthcoming. Counseling patients and their families remains somewhat controversial and limited, but is an important aspect of treatment. Practitioners need to remain current in their understanding and treatment of this disease, as new developments are frequent, and management is likely to change as this knowledge is considered and integrated into more optimal treatment algorithms.

References

Anhang, R., Goodman, A., & Goldie, S. J. (2004). HPV communication: Review of existing research and recommendations for patient education. *CA Cancer Journal for Clinicians, 54*(5), 248–259.

Chung, C. H., & Gillison, M. L. (2009). Human papillomavirus in head and neck cancer: Its role in pathogenesis and clinical implications. *Clinical Cancer Research, 15*(22), 6758–6762.

Conway, M. J., & Meyers, C. (2009) Replication and assembly of human papillomaviruses. *Journal of Dental Research, 88*(4), 307–317.

Fakhry, C., & Gillison, M. L. (2006) Clinical implications of human papillomavirus in head and neck cancers. *Journal of Clinical Oncology, 24*(17), 2606–2611.

Gillison, M. L. (2004) Human papillomavirus-associated head and neck cancer is a distinct epidemiologic, clinical, and molecular entity. *Seminars in Oncology, 31*(6),744–754.

Gillison, M. L., Chaturvedi, A. K., & Lowy, D. R. (2008) HPV prophylactic vaccines and the potential prevention of noncervical cancers in both men and women. *Cancer, 113*(10 Suppl.), 3036–3046.

Hennessey P. T., Westra, W. H., & Califano, J. A. (2009) Human papillomavirus and head and neck squamous cell carcinoma: Recent evidence and clinical implications. *Journal of Dental Research, 88*(4), 300–306.

Horvath, C. A., Boulet, G. A., Renoux , V. M., Delvenne, P. O., & Bogers, J. P. (2010). Mechanisms of cell entry by human papillomaviruses: An overview. *Virology Journal, 7*, 11.

Kreimer, A. R., Bhatia, R. K., Messeguer, A. L., González, P., Herrero, R., & Giuliano, A. R. (2010). Oral human papillomavirus in healthy individuals: A systematic review of the literature. *Sexually Transmitted Diseases, 37*(6), 386–391.

Marur, S., D'Souza, G., Westra, W. H., & Forastiere, A. A. (2010) HPV-associated head and neck cancer: A virus-related cancer epidemic. *Lancet Oncology, 11*(8), 781–789.

Stanley, M. (2010). Pathology and epidemiology of HPV infection in females. *Gynecologic Oncology, 117*(2 Suppl.), S5–S10.

Veldhuijzen, N. J., Snijders, P. J., Reiss, P., Meijer, C. J., & van de Wijgert, J. H. (2010) Factors affecting transmission of mucosal human papillomavirus. *Lancet Infectious Diseases, 10*(12), 862–874. Epub 2010 Nov 11.

3

MEETING THE CHALLENGES OF TREATMENT PLANNING AND SURGERY FOR CANCER OF THE HEAD AND NECK

Eugene N. Myers, MD, FACS, FRCS Edin (Hon)

PART I:
Determining Treatment for Oral and
Head and Neck Cancer

Squamous cell carcinoma arises from the surface cells of the skin and the mucous membrane which line the mouth, throat, and larynx (voice box) and is the most common form of cancer of the head and neck. Skin cancers (squamous cell, basal cell, and malignant melanoma) arise in response to long-term exposure to the sun. Skin cancer is also prevalent in patients who have received kidney transplants.

Squamous cell cancer of the mucous membrane usually occurs in individuals with a history of long-term tobacco and alcohol abuse. In recent years, evidence has shown that the human papilloma virus (HPV), which is known to be the cause of virtually all cervical cancers in women and may be the cause of cancer involving the tonsil and base of the tongue in nonsmokers. This information suggests that there may be two distinct pathways involved in the development of cancer of the tonsil and the base of the tongue, one driven by tobacco and alcohol abuse and the other induced by HPV, usually types 16 and 18 (D'Souza et al., 2007; see Chapter 2).

Other forms of cancer, such as malignant melanoma and adenocarcinoma, may arise from the mucous membranes of the mouth, nose, and sinuses. Lymphomas can occur in the palate, tonsil, base of the tongue, nasopharynx, or lymph nodes in the neck.

Cancer of the head and neck is often diagnosed at an advanced stage for several reasons. One is that the symptoms produced by cancer of the head and neck are similar to those associated with infections such as: sore throat, hoarseness, ear pain, nasal discharge, and swelling in the neck. Another reason for delay in diagnosis is that some patients are in denial about their symptoms, are overcome by fear, or are afraid to go to their doctor or dentist. Patients who do not seek treatment may manage their own symptoms for extended periods of time with various medications until the cancer is in an advanced stage (Ridge, Glisson, Horwitz, & Lango, 2005).

Individuals with cancer arising in the mucous membranes may present with a variety of symptoms depending on the structures involved. Patients with cancer of the vocal folds usually present with hoarseness. Other symptoms include: sore throat, difficulty swallowing, coughing up blood, and aspiration (food going into the windpipe with swallowing) (Ridge et al., 2005). Patients with advanced stage cancer may experience progressive shortness of breath or complete airway obstruction requiring placement of a breathing tube (tracheostomy).

Ear pain (otalgia) reflects "referred pain" secondary to cancer invading nerves of the throat, which also supply sensation to the ear. Because of the pain, some patients are mistakenly treated for an ear infection without having the thorough examination of the head and neck necessary to find the source of the pain.

Patients with cancer of the tongue or the floor of the mouth (the area under the tongue) complain of soreness, pain, bleeding, or ill-fitting dentures. This may progress to difficulty with swallowing accompanied by weight loss or with articulation (forming words). Some patients may complain of spitting out blood. Some may also have ear pain or a foul odor to the breath. In advanced cases the cancer may invade the muscles that open the mouth (trismus) leading to difficulty eating and weight loss.

Cancer of the tonsil and base of the tongue may present with sore throat and difficulty swallowing but some patients will not have any local symptoms, but rather may present with a lump in one or both sides of the neck. This lump represents spread (metastasis) of the cancer into the lymph nodes of the neck.

Nasopharyngeal cancer is usually seen in Asians and is rare in Caucasians. The most frequent symptoms include: hearing loss, nasal blockage, or a lump in the neck. In advanced cases, destruction of the base of the skull can cause symptoms related to loss of local nerve function.

When the patient's primary care physician (PCP) or dentist suspects cancer, the patient should be referred for performance of a biopsy (Ridge et al., 2005). Current treatment is often multidisciplinary in nature with patients treated by a team of doctors, but the surgeon is usually the captain of the team and is responsible for making appropriate referrals to other team members. These other members may include medical oncologists, radiation oncologists, oral maxillofacial surgeons, dentists, maxillofacial prosthodontists, nutritionists, social workers, psychiatrists, specialized nurses, speech and swallowing therapists, hospice, and clergy.

A comprehensive history should be taken in addition to local symptoms in the head and neck. Additionally, a recording of general health considerations (comorbidities), such as problems with heart, lungs, liver, diabetes, and HIV should be recorded. Addictions such as tobacco, alcohol, and narcotics must be revealed because, when present, these may have a profound effect on the immediate or long-term treatment program.

A thorough physical examination must include the skin, mouth, larynx (voice box), throat, nasopharynx, and neck. Tumor diagrams should be used to record the location and size of the tumor. The neck must be thoroughly examined to detect lymph nodes that may contain cancer. The head and neck surgeon must evaluate the extent of invasion below the surface into the deep tissues. The teeth and gums must be examined because patients who smoke and drink heavily may also have poor dentition and gum (periodontal) disease. A flexible tube with a light on the tip (endoscope) may be placed through the nose to examine the throat and larynx in detail and to take photos. This procedure is called flexible endoscopy.

To fully evaluate the areas involved by the cancer, imaging studies such as ultrasound, CT scan, or MRI may be necessary. The use of PET-CT scan has become popular for initial staging purposes and then later to reevaluate the patient, especially those who have received chemoradiation therapy (Fukui, Blodgett, Snyderman, Johnson, & Myers, 2005). These studies are done on an outpatient basis and usually involve an intravenous injection of contrast fluid, which helps the radiologist to evaluate the areas of interest. On the basis of physical examination and/or the scan, a fine-needle aspiration biopsy (FNAB) of a lump in the neck may be necessary to obtain a sample of cells for analysis. This may be done in either the doctor's office or the hospital, with ultrasound guidance. Cancer of the skin, lip, or mouth may be biopsied in the surgeon's office under local anesthesia. As most squamous cell carcinomas are ulcerated and have a poor blood supply, this procedure should be safe.

Once the evaluation is complete, the cancer is "staged" or classified according to certain criteria, including the size of the primary tumor (T) and depth of invasion, whether any lymph nodes (N) appear to be involved with cancer, and any evidence of distant spread (metastases [M]) (Gluckman & Wolfe, 2006). The TNM system is helpful in choosing treatment options and predicting prognosis.

Patients with cancer of the mucous membranes of the head and neck should have an endoscopic examination (endoscopy) and biopsy under general anesthesia. This allows a thorough evaluation without the usual gagging or discomfort (or both) associated with examination in the doctor's office. A preliminary examination by the patient's family doctor or hospital anesthesiologist will determine the patient's suitability to undergo the examination under anesthesia. An EKG, chest x-ray, and laboratory data are obtained and the patient's condition is optimized prior to anesthesia to prevent complications. The endoscopy also will help to determine the presence of other cancers in the lungs or in the esophagus that must be incorporated into the treatment program. Patients with bad teeth and gum infection should have dental extractions to promote better healing and to avoid complications after surgery and radiation.

The question of whether cancer of the head and neck should be treated by surgery alone, surgery followed by radiation therapy, surgery followed by radiation therapy and chemotherapy, or radiation with or without chemotherapy can be confusing to the patient. Patients must be informed in detail of all options: including no treatment, in certain cases.

When the patient is contemplating surgery, a thorough discussion with the surgeon is necessary to explain the risks and benefits of the procedure. This discussion should also include whether the surgery is performed as an outpatient or inpatient and the approximate length of hospital stay. Any surgical reconstruction usually is carried out immediately following the removal of the cancer and should be discussed because this increases the length of time of the procedure and the hospital stay. Patients with serious medical problems such as chronic lung disease or heart problems may be predisposed to serious postoperative complications.

Discharge planning is essential and important and ideally requires strong family support; however, this may not always be possible. In such cases discharge to an appropriate short-term care facility is essential. In certain cases, prolonged rehabilitation may be necessary. If this phase of the treatment program is not carefully planned, a growing sense of despair and stress may develop in the patient and lead to a frank depression, making the completion of therapy and reentry into society difficult (Gluckman & Wolfe, 2006). Issues such as pain management and adequate nutritional support also must be addressed.

PART II:
Surgical Procedures for Specific Oral and Head and Neck Cancers

The extent of surgery for cancer of the head and neck cancer depends on the size and the location of the primary cancer and the presence or absence of cancer in the neck. Early cancers such as those limited to the vocal cords (T1) are often treated with a laser. This brief operation is carried out in the operating room with the patient under general anesthesia on an outpatient basis. No pain is involved, although some muscle soreness in the shoulder and the back of the neck may be expected. Patients are usually required to rest their voice and to be on acid reflux medication to ensure good healing.

Patients with more locally advanced cancer of the larynx may be treated with "conservation surgery" (Johnson, 2008). These voice-sparing procedures are done through an incision in the neck with the intent of preserving the voice. A tracheostomy (a temporary opening in the trachea (windpipe) is required and remains in place for several weeks to allow for swelling of the remaining larynx to subside. Intravenous fluids are given for the first few days, after which nutrition is delivered through a tube usually placed directly into the stomach by way of a gastrostomy tube. Once the patient can breathe sufficiently with the tracheostomy tube plugged, the tracheostomy tube can be removed. Swallowing rehabilitation can then be started with the help of a speech-language pathologist or swallowing coach (dysphagia coach). Once patients can swallow and maintain their nutritional status, the feeding tube can be removed. In some cases tube feeding may continue after discharge. Patients who progress more slowly may be discharged to a skilled nursing facility. The surgeon should then follow up with the patient in his or her office, remove the gastrostomy and tracheostomy tubes at the appropriate time, and proceed with swallowing therapy. Pressure to discharge patients as early as possible will result in a modification of this plan, with the discharge likely to take place within the first few days and tube removal and swallowing therapy done on an outpatient basis. Patients undergoing laser surgery for more advanced cancer usually do not require a tracheotomy or insertion of a feeding tube. The quality of life following these surgical procedures to conserve the voice is usually good.

Robotic surgery (transoral robotic surgery or TORS) is now used in certain types of surgery for cancer of the head and neck. Weinstein and his team at the University of Pennsylvania quoted their experience in 225 cases performed using the robotic (TORS) technique (Weinstein, O'Malley, Desai, & Quon, 2009). They reported that this technique is feasible as it provides access to almost any cancer in the throat and mouth as well as many cancers in the larynx. The operations were found to be safe and no patient operated on by this technique required a blood transfusion. The functional outcome was excellent with 96% of their patients swallowing without the use of a feeding tube. This new surgical technique allows for better preservation of normal tissues and a potential for a decrease in the dose of postoperative radiation therapy (see Chapter 4).

A total laryngectomy is advised for patients who have locally advanced cancer, which makes it impossible to save any part of the larynx. A neck dissection usually is included. The same applies to patients who have gone through a full course of radiation therapy or chemotherapy in whom the treatment was not successful. Although a small number of these patients may be eligible for conservation surgery to preserve the voice, elderly patients or those who have poor lung function or severe cardiovascular disease are usually advised to have the entire larynx removed (total laryngectomy). Although conservation surgery may be technically feasible, the patient may lack the will or the strength to be successfully rehabilitated and may become dependent on the tracheostomy tube and a stomach tube for feeding due to the difficulty in swallowing caused by surgical removal of certain structures in the larynx essential for swallowing. The quality of life under these circumstances is not as good as with a total laryngectomy.

After a total laryngectomy, the throat muscles are sewn together to form a tube so that the patient can swallow normally. Preoperative radiation therapy changes the quality of the tissues and may result in delayed healing. Sometimes the edges of the swallowing passage may partially separate, producing leakage of saliva into the neck with resultant infection draining to the outside, forming a *fistula*. Small fistulas are treated by packing medicated gauze into the opening until the tissues heal completely and the leakage stops. Preoperative radiation therapy and malnutrition increase the fistula rate significantly. All patients with a fistula have a prolonged hospital course. A larger fistula or prolonged leak often requires surgical reconstruction (Tsou et al., 2010).

After the larynx has been removed, a small opening is made in the back wall of the trachea into the food passage and a rubber tube is inserted. This tube is removed approximately 2 weeks later after healing has taken place and a speaking valve is inserted. This enables the patient to speak when the hole in the neck (stoma) is covered with the thumb. Some surgeons prefer to puncture the windpipe and insert the valve at a later date (Eibling, 2008).

Once the tissue is sufficiently healed, patients may resume their usual activities with a good quality of life. A stoma cover may be used during the day and can be obtained along with other comfort items by contacting the Web site of the International Association of Laryngectomees (IAL) at http://www.larynxlink.com.

The pharynx (throat) surrounds the larynx. Cancers that arise in this area may require removal of all or part of the larynx and surrounding throat tissue. Removal of the larynx requires surgical reconstruction to permit swallowing. Several choices are available to accomplish this. A flap of skin or muscle from the chest, which includes its own arteries and veins, is folded to form a tube and sewn to the remaining tissue of the throat. In more recent years, an alternative approach has been developed using a "free flap" or "free tissue transfer" in which skin from the forearm or thigh or a portion of the small intestine (jejunum) is transferred together with its own arteries and veins and sewn into the remaining parts of the throat (Wong & Wei, 2010). The arteries and veins of the free flap are sewn to the arteries and veins in the neck. If a free flap from the forearm is used, a skin graft is used to resurface the donor site. Provision for the insertion of a voice valve is also included at the time of surgery. Once the swelling has subsided the patient can swallow, which is one of the most important aspects in measuring the quality of life in a laryngectomy patient.

Oral cancer can affect the tongue (the most common site), the floor of the mouth, the gums, the roof of the mouth (palate), and the jawbone (mandible). Radiation therapy without chemotherapy usually does not play a role in the primary treatment of oral cancers for cure but may be used postoperatively. A neck dissection usually is included at the time of the removal of the cancer, regardless of whether the lymph nodes are enlarged.

Cancer of the tongue almost always arises on the side of the tongue. Surgery to remove a small cancer (partial glossectomy) will also include excision of some surrounding normal tissue to ensure complete tumor removal and allow for closure of the cut edges of the tongue with a few stitches. A pathologist examines the edges of the tissues to be certain that all cancer cells have been removed. This procedure does not require a tracheostomy or a feeding tube. Patients begin to swallow the night of the surgery and usually are discharged 1 or 2 days later once the neck dissection is healed sufficiently. Normal speech and swallowing are to be expected.

Removal of more extensive cancer of the tongue may require a skin graft. The graft is usually taken from the thigh and sewn into the edges of the tongue defect. A thin, pliable free flap from the forearm is an alternative. A tracheostomy is performed and a nasogastric feeding tube is used. In 5 to 7 days, the tubes are removed and the patient can be discharged.

When cancer occurs in the back part (base) of the tongue, it may be necessary to divide the jawbone in the midline to provide enough room to see and remove the entire cancer. The jawbone is then repaired using small metal plates and screws. A more direct approach to the base of the tongue involves going through the neck above the larynx and removing the cancer.

The entire tongue is removed only in cases in which the entire tongue is involved with tumor. Patients must be in general good health and have good lung function to survive this surgery and have a reasonable quality of life afterward. In such cases, the entire tongue is removed (total glossectomy) along with bilateral neck dissections. A feeding tube is usually inserted into the stomach (PEG or "G" tube) to provide access to nourishment while patients are healing and subsequently learning how to swallow. Following surgery, patients are restricted to a thick liquid and pureed diet. The tracheostomy tube is later plugged but kept in place until the patient is swallowing without aspiration, at which time the tracheostomy tube can be removed. Patients with poor lung function cannot tolerate this procedure and also will require a total laryngectomy along with removal of the tongue to avoid developing aspiration pneumonia. Reconstruction with tissue flaps is required in these advanced cases.

Cancer of the floor of the mouth usually occurs in the midline region. These cancers are usually removed through the mouth. If the cancer is in the midline, both sides of the neck are dissected. If the cancer is limited to one side, only the neck on that side of the cancer is dissected. If the cancer is very close to or adherent to the jawbone, the bone of the gum (and teeth) must be removed. After removal, the tissues are examined by the pathologist to be certain that all of the cancer has been removed. The raw surfaces are then reconstructed using a skin graft or a free flap taken from the forearm (radial forearm free flap). The graft is sewn into the defect, and a gauze packing is applied. A tracheostomy and nasogastric (NG) feeding tube are inserted and removed within 5 to 7 days. Patients should be able to speak and swallow normally when the healing is complete.

The jawbone (mandible) may be invaded by cancer directly from the soft tissues of the gum or secondarily by cancer of the floor of the mouth or tongue. In advanced cases the skin of the lip, chin, or cheek may also be involved. The approach is usually through an incision in the skin rather than just through the mouth. Neck dissections are always included with this surgery. It is important to remove adequate amounts of what looks like normal bone adjacent to the cancer as the pathologist cannot examine the bone margin under the microscope by frozen section at the time of surgery. After removal of the jawbone and necessary skin or tissue of the mouth, reconstruction is carried out. This is particularly true in patients in whom the bone supporting the chin is involved because failure to reconstruct this area leads to inability to close the mouth, speak, or swallow. The introduction of free tissue flaps containing bone from either the arm or leg allows for reconstruction of the jawbone. Metal plates and screws are used to attach the bone graft to the remaining unaffected jawbone (Wong & Wei, 2010). Tracheostomy and an NG tube are used and are removed once the swelling subsides and the tissues are healed.

Small cancers of the inside of the cheek may be removed through the mouth and a skin graft is used to resurface the raw area. A gauze pack holds the skin graft in place. A neck dissection is included. No tracheostomy or NG tube is necessary in such cases. Patients with more advanced cancers in the cheek may require removal of the overlying skin or jawbone when involved. This requires reconstruction as described previously, with resumption of normal speaking and swallowing expected along with a good quality of life.

Cancer of the roof of the mouth (hard palate) and upper gum is usually squamous cell carcinoma, although cancers (adenocarcinomas) may also arise from minor salivary glands or mucous glands in this area. The cancer may invade the underlying bone, which must be removed. In these circumstances, separation between the mouth and nose is lost, resulting in food exiting through the nose when swallowing and less intelligible speech.

Prior to this type of surgery, the patient must be referred to a maxillofacial prosthodontist (a dentist with special training in making dental appliances, or prostheses) to design and construct a prosthesis to replace the roof of the mouth, restore oral-nasal separation, and allow for normal speech and swallowing. Patients with remaining upper teeth will have a prosthesis (obturator) that clips onto the teeth. Patients without teeth have a more difficult time with retention of the prosthesis due to the weight of the denture. Patients with more extensive cancer requiring removal of the surrounding soft tissue, such as the soft palate and tonsil, will benefit from the prosthesis, but speech and swallowing will not completely return to normal, but will be intelligible.

After healing has progressed, a "temporary prosthesis" (without teeth) is made while the tissues heal further to accommodate a permanent prosthesis with teeth. Daily oral cleansing with salt water or hydrogen peroxide mixed in equal amounts of water is very useful. A water pick may be used to keep the cavity free of dried mucus.

In recent years techniques for palatal reconstruction using free flaps containing bone have been devised to eliminate the need for prostheses and to close the surgical defect (Wong & Wei, 2010). On the positive side, a prosthesis is not necessary; on the negative side, the cavity is no longer open for the surgeon to examine and monitor for possible recurrence of the cancer. Some of this risk is eliminated with the use of scanning imaging techniques including MRI and PET scans.

Cancer of the head and neck has the potential to spread (metastasize) to the lymph nodes in the neck and a radical neck dissection may be necessary. This procedure consists of removal of all of the lymph nodes in the neck, the jugular vein, the large muscle (sternocleidomastoid) in the neck, and the spinal accessory nerve which supplies innervation to the shoulder muscle (trapezius).

Although control of active cancer of the lymph nodes is excellent with this operation, especially when combined with postoperative radiation and possibly chemotherapy, there are drawbacks to this procedure, including altered cosmetic appearance, reduced shoulder function, and decreased range of arm motion. Patients who have had a radical neck dissection must enter into a physical therapy program, specifically designed to prevent shoulder dysfunction. A diligent exercise program will allow the patient to avoid shoulder pain, marked disability, and a severe cosmetic defect.

In more recent years, the concept of the "selective neck dissection," rather than observation or radical dissection, has become popular (Schmitz, Machiels, Weynard, Gregoire, & Hamoir, 2009). This operation can be performed in patients without obvious positive lymph nodes. As only the lymph nodes are removed, the patient's normal appearance and function are preserved. If cancer is found, additional treatment with radiation therapy or combined chemoradiation may be given. If all lymph nodes are free of cancer, no further treatment may be necessary and the patient's chance for cure is better. Patients who have had a selective neck dissection usually have minimal side effects. The selective neck dissection also may be used for patients with limited cancer in the lymph nodes.

Cancer involving the parotid gland is relatively rare. The parotid gland, which produces saliva, is located just in front of and below the ear and usually is associated with benign tumors

(80 to 90%). The characteristic sign of a tumor in the parotid gland is a painless lump or mass. It is difficult to tell benign from malignant on physical examination; however, if the mass has grown rapidly, is associated with pain and/or paralysis of the face, it is almost always malignant.

Low-grade cancer of the parotid gland is treated by surgical removal through an incision in front of and below the ear. The facial nerve usually can be preserved, whereas neck dissection is not necessary and the quality of life should be undisturbed.

Patients with high-grade cancer of the parotid gland, especially if facial paralysis is present, will need a total parotidectomy, removal of the facial nerve, facial nerve reconstruction, and a neck dissection followed by radiation therapy (Laramore, 2007).

Patients with cancer of the head and neck are under great emotional strain during this time because the cancer that threatens their lives and the operations, designed to cure the cancer, also may threaten the patients' appearance and function. The first few days after surgery, the patients usually are quite happy and, in fact, elated and relieved to realize that, despite the usual fears that they will die under anesthesia, they find that they have survived. However, 3 to 4 days postoperatively, it is not unusual for patients to become depressed. This may be due to the realization that they have cancer and that its treatment will impact their lifestyle. Their emotional stress may be magnified by the loss of interpersonal support systems and the obvious loss, whether temporary or permanent, of the ability to communicate (Lydiatt, 2006). Recognition of this problem by the surgeon; a frank discussion of the fact that this is a natural postoperative event; and a positive attitude on the part of the surgeons, the nursing staff, and the personal caregiver often alleviate these temporary symptoms of depression without the need for medications or psychiatric consultation.

The diagnosis of cancer instantly changes the life of the individual. However, a word should be said about the caregivers. The patient's loved ones and caregivers may experience emotions similar to those of the patient. They may worry not only about the patient's survival, appearance, and function but also about financial security and how the patient's disability may affect future plans. They even may become preoccupied with thoughts of death. Although a patient experiences the pain of surgery and other forms of cancer treatment, caregivers have a shared pain for the impact of the treatment on the patient and also on their family's structure, lifestyle, and future. There is a need for the entire support system to come into play to cope with these problems (Gluckman & Wolfe, 2006).

Current management involves treatment by a team of professionals. The surgeon, who is usually the first to meet the patient, should be the one to monitor the patient's overall progress. Follow-up visits should be frequent enough to answer the patient's questions about symptoms, including pain, lack of normal function, dry mouth from radiation therapy, or need for further treatment or rehabilitation. Close follow-up is also necessary because of the potential for patients with squamous cell carcinoma to develop second primary cancers (15 to 20%) throughout their lifetime. Second primary cancers may occur in the head and neck, lung, or esophagus and are more frequent in patients who do not stop smoking. Continued surveillance is required to diagnose second primary cancer at the earliest possible stage.

Surgeons and their staffs must be aware not only of the physical needs, such as nutrition and pain relief, but also of the emotional needs of the patient and the caregiver and the impact on the family unit. They should be willing, able, and available to meet their needs and to provide support.

References

D'Souza, G., Kreimer, A., Viscidi, R., Pawlita, M., Fakhry, C., Koch, W. M., . . . Gillison, M. L. (2007). Case-control study of human papillomavirus and oropharyngeal cancer. *New England Journal of Medicine, 356*, 1944–1956.

Eibling, D. E. (2008). Voice restoration after total laryngectomy. In E. N. Myers (Ed.), *Operative otolaryngology—head and neck surgery*. Philadelphia, PA: Saunders/Elsevier.

Fukui, M. D., Blodgett, T. M., Snyderman, C. H., Johnson, J. T., & Myers, E. N. (2005). Combined PET-CT in the head and neck: Part II, Diagnostic uses and pitfalls of oncologic imaging. *Radio Graphics, 25,* 913–930.

Gluckman, J. L., & Wolfe, M. (2006). Head and neck cancer in the geriatric patient. In K. H. Calhoun, & D. E. Eibling (Eds.), *Geriatric otolaryngology*. New York, NY: Taylor & Francis.

Johnson, J. T. (2008). Horizontal partial laryngectomy; Postoperative management. In E. N. Myers (Ed.), *Operative otolaryngology—head and neck surgery*. Philadelphia, PA: Saunders/Elsevier.

Laramore, G. E. (2007). Role of radiotherapy in the treatment of tumors of the salivary glands. In E. N. Myers & R. L. Ferris (Eds.), *Salivary gland disorders*. Berlin, Heidelberg, Germany: Springer-Verlag.

Lydiatt, W. M. (2006, September). A review of depression in head and neck cancer. *News from SPOHNC.*

Ridge, J. A., Glisson, B. S., Horwitz, E. M., & Lango, M. N. (2005). Head and neck tumors. In R. Pazdur, W. Hoskins, L. Coia, & L. Wagman (Eds.), *Cancer management: A multidisciplinary approach*. Manhasset, NY: Oncology Publishing Group.

Schmitz, S., Machiels, J. P., Weynand, B., Gregoire, V., & Hamoir, M. (2009). Results of selective neck dissection in the primary management of head and neck squamous cell carcinoma. *European Archives Otorhinolaryngology, 266,* 437–443.

Tsou, Y-A., Hua, C-H., Lin, M-H., Tseng, H-C., Tsai, M-H., & Shaha, A. (2010). Comparison of pharyngocutaneous fistula between patients followed by primary laryngopharyngectomy and salvage laryngopharyngectomy for advanced hypopharyngeal cancer. *Head and Neck, 32,* 1494–1500.

Weinstein, G., O'Malley, B., Desai, S., Quon, H. (2009). Transoral robotic surgery: Does the ends justify the means? *Current Opinion in Otolaryngology and Head and Neck Surgery, 17,* 126–131.

Wong, C-H., & Wei, F-C. (2010). Microsurgical free flap in head and neck reconstruction. *Head and Neck, 32,* 1236–1245.

4

MEETING THE CHALLENGES OF TRANSORAL ROBOTIC SURGERY (TORS)

Gregory S. Weinstein, MD
Bert W. O'Malley, Jr, MD

Introduction

This chapter introduces the reader to TransOral Robotic Surgery (TORS), which utilizes the da Vinci® surgical system to allow for minimally invasive surgery for patients with benign and malignant tumors of the head and neck. TORS is actually a group of several minimally invasive procedures that are useful for a wide variety of benign and malignant conditions. Nonetheless, the most common indication for TORS is for advanced oropharyngeal carcinoma (AOC).

TORS was developed in the context of two important trends related to oropharyngeal carcinoma. The first has been the increased use of chemoradiation in the management of AOC and the increase in severe side effects associated with this treatment. The second important trend has been the changing causes of AOC with a decline in smoking-related cancers and the increase in the number of human papillomavirus (HPV)-related AOC.

Advancements over the past decade in the nonsurgical treatment for head and neck cancer utilizing radiation and chemotherapy have resulted in avoiding surgical removal of portions of the throat and neck, but not without severe oral complications. Unfortunately, more than 80% of patients with oropharyngeal cancers present with advanced stages of disease. A recent analysis of the United States national cancer database by Chen, Schrag, Hao, Stewart, and Ward (2007) revealed an increase in the use of combined chemoradiation for the treatment of advanced oropharyngeal carcinoma (AOC) during the period 1985 to 2001. The rationale behind the increased use of chemoradiation for AOC has been to improve survival and local control compared to radiation therapy alone, and to improve functional and quality of life (QOL) outcomes compared to "radical open surgical approaches."

Forestiere (1999), a medical oncologist and an expert in the use of chemoradiation for head and neck cancers, acknowledged that "preservation of the organ does not equate to preservation of function. Severe and chronic mucosal injury and tissue fibrosis as a late toxic effect of intensive radiochemotherapy regimens may leave patients with poor swallowing function and thus be dependent on a gastrostomy tube."

Increasing numbers of studies demonstrate that one of the key challenges in the treatment of AOC with chemotherapy and radiation is the potential for long-term swallowing problems requiring gastrostomy tube. Indeed, three recent studies evaluating state of the art chemotherapy-intensity modulated radiation therapy (CIMRT) in the treatment of AOC reported permanent percutaneous endoscopic gastrostomy (PEG) rates between 9 and 38% (Lawson et al., 2008).

Several groups of researchers have found that permanent PEG dependence is one of the strongest clinical predictors of QOL in head and neck cancer patients (Terrell et al., 2004). Consequently, the key challenge of treating patients with advanced head and neck cancer is avoiding the significant impact of long-term swallowing problems without compromising treatment outcome, and meeting this challenge was one of the key reasons for the development of TransOral Robotic Surgery (TORS).

A second trend that has paralleled the increased use of chemoradiation for oropharyngeal carcinoma has been the dramatic decrease in the number of smoking-related cancers and the rise in the number of HPV-related oropharyngeal cancers. The most common areas of the throat for HPV cancers to arise in are the tongue base and the tonsillar areas, which together account for the vast majority of oropharyngeal cancers. In our recent study, 75% of patients with AOC were HPV related (Cohen, Weinstein, O'Malley, Feldman, & Quon, 2011). The United States Centers for Disease Control (2011) has noted that the number of HPV-related head and neck cancer is now approaching the number of HPV-related cancers of the cervix (Lawson et al., 2008). In HPV-related cancers of the cervix, where there is early diagnosis via pap smear, physicians are able to find these cancers very early (Berkowitz, Saraiya, Benard, & Yabroff., 2010). However, there is no Pap-smear equivalent for early diagnosis of HPV-related oropharyngeal carcinoma and, therefore, the vast majority of these cancers have already spread to neck lymph nodes at the time of diagnosis, thus representing an advanced stage cancer. In addition, evidence is mounting that nonsmoking patients with HPV-related cancers who are treated with chemoradiation have better cure rates than patients with either HPV-negative cancers or HPV-positive cancers in patients with a history of smoking who are treated with chemoradiation (Kumar et al., 2007).This has led many clinicians to recommend that patients with HPV-related advanced oropharyngeal carcinoma undergo chemoradiation. This in turn has led to a number of functional and oncologic problems.

First, some clinicians may lump all HPV-related cancers as one group and advocate chemoradiation for all HPV-related cancers regardless of the size of the cancer and the smoking history of the patient. This trend is problematic as it is known that a patient who has a history of smoking, as well as HPV positivity will not have the very high cure rates that are seen in the HPV nonsmoker. In addition, although most HPV-related cancers are early T stage (T1 and T2), meaning that the cancers are fairly small in the tonsil or tongue base where they began, some are larger T4 cancers. There is evidence that these larger cancers do not have as high a cure rate following chemoradiation even if they are HPV positive (Sedaghat et al., 2009).

We thus know that the present standard of high intensity chemoradiation for AOC results in a large percentage of patients needing a lifelong stomach tube for feeding. Given the relatively younger age that patients with HPV positive cancers present compared to smokers' cancers, and the higher cure rates, many of these young patients are destined to live a longer post-treatment period with poor QOL related to swallowing.

TransOral Robotic Surgery (TORS) and the Management of Advanced Oropharyngeal Carcinoma

In 2004, in an effort to deal with devastating swallowing problems that we were observing for many patients undergoing chemoradiation for cancers of the head and neck a translational research program in TransOral Robotic Surgery (TORS) was begun at the University of Pennsylvania. Although other minimally invasive techniques had existed for decades utilizing transoral laser approaches, these techniques were widely applied to early laryngeal (voice box) cancers, but were very difficult to apply to the tongue base and tonsil due to difficulty with surgical access, visualization and instrumentation issues and hence were only done by a small group of experts (Grant et al., 2006). Our hope was to create a group of minimally invasive surgical procedures that would allow avoidance or de-intensification of postoperative radiation and chemoradiation and thus improve swallowing outcomes. The goal of this preclinical research program was to see if minimally invasive surgical procedures could be accomplished via the mouth using the da Vinci® surgical system (Intuitive Surgical, Inc, Sunnyvale, CA) with the ultimate plan of sharing these new procedures with members of the head and neck surgical community

A series of experiments in mannequin, animal, and cadaver models proved the feasibility of this approach (Hockstein, O'Malley, & Weinstein., 2005, 2006; O'Malley et al., 2006a). Thus in May of 2005 the first patient research in TORS was begun at the University of Pennsylvania. During the first year of the clinical trial, new surgical techniques for cancers of the larynx, tongue base and tonsil were offered to patients and reported on in the literature (O'Malley et al., 2006b, Weinstein, O'Malley, Snyder, & Hockenstein, 2007; Weinstein, O'Malley, Snyder, Sherman, & Quon, 2007).

In October, 2006 in a spirit of collaboration and in an effort to expand clinical research in this fledgling field the two authors of this chapter led a research training session for 11 invited surgeons. This research training course included lectures, with cadaver demonstrations followed by cadaver dissections by the participants. Their research protocol was shared with all 12 surgeons who participated. Most of these surgeons utilized this training successfully and many of them published articles about their experience with TORS, providing clear evidence that this research training session was a success. The results of these studies and efforts led to the U.S. Food and Drug Administration (FDA) clearing the use of the da Vinci® surgical system for transoral surgery in December of 2009.

Traditional Surgical Alternatives for the Management of Oropharyngeal Carcinoma

The conventional primary surgical approach for higher stage T3 and T4 stage AOC has been open radical surgical approaches, frequently requiring opening the jaw to gain access for resection. These open radical approaches have much greater morbidity associated with them compared to transoral surgery (O'Brien et al., 1998). The technique requires, in many cases, splitting the jaw or transecting the pharynx via the neck for access, placement of a temporary, or in some cases, a permanent tracheotomy (breathing tube in the windpipe placed with a neck incision), prolonged operations (8 to 12 hours), prolonged hospitalizations (6 to10 days), and finally a long period of severe dysphagia (difficulty swallowing), which can result in permanent placement of a PEG. Although transoral laser microsurgery (TLM) was introduced decades ago, the main application has been in the resection of larynx cancer, with only two series being published on TLM for tongue base resection and none on TLM tonsillar carcinoma resection (Grant et al., 2006).

Why Is There Such a Problem for Transoral Resection of the Very Back Part of the Tongue?

Traditional transoral surgery can, at times, be surgically awkward secondary to: (1) the instruments (many of which were conceptualized in the 19th century), which are long and of limited functionality and passed through long tubular laryngoscopes that limit the view of the operative field; (2) the microscopic optics, which are outside the oral cavity; and (3) the laser, which is a "line of sight" beam far from the lesion as well as tangential to the tongue base lesions that is being resected, whereas transoral approaches using conventional technologies do exist and cause less "surgical damage" than open radical surgical resections, so far only a few surgeons have reported on these technologies, which in our opinion is because of the limited surgical access obtained with existing instrumentation. TORS has overcome the limitations that have been seen in the past with other nonrobotic transoral resection approaches.

How Is TransOral Robotic Surgery (TORS) Done?

The da Vinci® Robotic Surgical System consists of three basic components: a surgeon's console, a patient cart with articulated or multijointed mechanical arms, and sterilizable instruments. The console includes a computer, video monitor, and instrument controls, and is located in the operating room adjacent to the operating room table. The console is connected via computer to the "patient cart" which has mechanical arms holding the endoscope (surgical TV camera) and sterile surgical tools (e.g., forceps, scissors, electrocautery, etc.). These arms are located immediately adjacent to the patient on the operating room table. The surgeon sits at the console and controls the position and movement of the arms and surgical tools. The design of these tools is based upon well-established, commonly used surgical instruments. The da Vinci® Robotic Surgical System is a "manual image-guided surgery" system that is computer *enhanced* rather than "computer *guided* robotic surgery."

Use of this system in the aforementioned configuration facilitates a motion-scaled translation of the surgeon's hand and finger movements at the console to precise and tremor-free movements of the arms and instruments. Its advantages include:

1. The importance of using "mouth gags" rather than laryngoscopes to pass the robotic arms transorally,
2. The optimal position of the "patient cart" to the operative bed to allow for successful placement of robotic arms transorally,
3. Best practices to ensure safety and efficacy, and
4. The critical role of the bedside assistant during TORS (i.e., suctioning, retraction, application hemoclips).

A major distinction between transoral laser microsurgery and TORS is that laser surgery is done by cutting up the malignant tumor into small pieces whereas TORS, as taught to the vast majority of surgeons, is done with the robotic electrocautery tool and the entire cancer is removed as one piece. Although some authors have experimented with laser coupled with the robot during TORS, the vast majority of reports in the literature use the standard approach without the laser, and at this time the laser coupled with TORS is not the approach recommended by the authors of this chapter.

TransOral Robotic Surgery Improves Swallowing Outcomes

A recent study at the University of Pennsylvania of a subset of the original cohort of patients who underwent TORS for AOC, showed a dramatic decrease in the number of PEG-dependent patients when compared to similar reports in the literature for chemoradiation (O'Brien et al., 1998). The primary objectives of this study were to:

1. Determine the oncologic outcomes, with a minimum of 18 months follow-up, of 47 patients with AOC treated with TORS, neck dissection, and adjuvant radiation with or without chemotherapy, as indicated,
2. Assess the rate of PEG dependence for patients who were followed for a minimum of 1 year post-treatment, and
3. Assess safety and efficacy endpoints of this novel strategy.

There were three key findings identified. The first is that our novel TORS approach for AOC resulted in comparable oncologic outcomes as compared to published chemoradiation reports with disease-specific survival of 90% at 2 years and local, regional, and distant failure rates comparable to the state of the art nonsurgical alternative, chemotherapy IMRT (de Arruda et al., 2006; Lawson et al., 2008). Of note, none of the cases reported in our study required complex free flap reconstruction, which is a major benefit to patients. Of the many hundreds of TORS cases reported to date in the literature, only a handful have been reported with free flap reconstruction. Thus, at the present time, free flaps are recommended only in very selected cases, for instance, in patients who undergo TORS following chemoradiation failure.

Second, the low rate (2.1%) at which cancer was left at the surgical margins (i.e., positive margin rate) coupled with the pathologic findings of the lymph nodes, which were removed during a nonrobotic neck dissection (i.e., removal of involved or at risk lymph nodes in the neck, most often with a nonradical approach) allowed for pathologic stratification or categorization and de-intensification of the treatment with 10.6% of patients avoiding radiation and chemotherapy, and 38.3% of patients avoiding chemotherapy.

The third and most exciting finding was an unexpectedly low PEG dependency rate of only 2.4%, which is much lower than the reported PEG dependency for the state of the art nonsurgical alternative, chemotherapy and IMRT (9 to 38%) (Lawson et al., 2008, Rusthoven et al., 2008).

TORS Training Ensures Access for Patients

From the outset, our goal in TORS-related clinical research has been to teach other teams these techniques and to allow for further research to be done elsewhere; and also to prove the principle of "teachability" of the TORS technique. The research training seminar, held in 2006 at the University of Pennsylvania, brought surgeons from around the United States together for a day-long training session to learn the TORS techniques, share practice concepts, and begin discussions for collaborative research. This training program was a great success and resulted in active TORS clinical programs in numerous institutions in the United States. Since FDA clearance in 2009, Post-Graduate Certification was created at the University of Pennsylvania. Recently, a similar course was created at the M.D. Anderson Hospital in

Houston, Texas. Over 100 practicing surgeons have attended the training, which includes online learning, animal lab, surgeon-led cadaver training lab, case observation, and proctorship. In addition to Post-Graduate Certification, this year (2011) the Society of Robotic Surgery began certifying fellowship programs. The goal here is to ensure that recent graduates from training also have the opportunity to learn these important techniques.

The Society of Robotic Surgery (SRS) (http://www.srobotics .org) is the largest robotic surgery society with over 400 members and the board of this society has taken on the responsibility of certifying fellowship training in robotics across specialties. At present, the only programs eligible for SRS TORS certification are fellows who are enrolled in the American Head and Neck Society Advanced Head and Neck Surgery training fellowships. Patients considering robotic surgery as a treatment option should discuss overall experience and certification with their TORS surgeons.

Summary: TransOral Robotic Surgery (TORS) Is Useful for a Variety of Tumors and Anatomic Sites

TORS has been very helpful for patients with oropharyngeal cancer and has provided an excellent alternative to high intensity chemoradiation. This has been of major significance given the HPV epidemic and its impact on the increasing numbers of HPV-related oropharyngeal cancers today. Nonetheless, TORS has been shown to be excellent for other anatomic sites and benign and malignant tumors as well.

A number of reports have shown the value of TORS for larynx cancers that involve the supraglottis (Alon, Kasparbauer, Olsen, & Moore., 2011). Dr. William Wei underwent Postgraduate TORS Certification at the University of Pennsylvania and returned to Hong Kong and created a new TORS procedure for the resection of recurrent nasopharyngeal carcinoma (Yin Tsang,

Ho, & Wei., 2011). Although TORS is best used in patients prior to chemoradiation, a number of reports have shown the value of TORS for cancers that have recurred following radiation and chemoradiation (Dean et al., 2010). TORS has also been shown to be of value in avoiding neck incisions and jaw splitting procedures during the removal of parapharyngeal space tumors. New surgical applications continues to be developed for TORS (O'Malley., et al., 2010; Weinstein et al., 2010).

References

Alon E. E., Kasperbauer, J. L., Olsen, K. D., & Moore, E. J. (2011). Feasibility of transoral robotic-assisted supraglottic laryngectomy. *Head and Neck*, Apr 15. doi: 10.1002/hed.21719.

Berkowitz, Z., Saraiya, M., Benard, V., & Yabroff, K. R. (2010). Common abnormal results of pap and human papillomavirus cotesting: What physicians are recommending for management. *Obstetrics and Gyncecology, 116*(6), 1332–1340.

Chen A. Y., Schrag, N., Hao, Y., Stewart, A., & Ward, E. (2007). Changes in treatment of advanced oropharyngeal cancer, 1985–2001. *Laryngoscope, 117*(1), 16–21.

Cohen, M. A., Weinstein, G. S., O'Malley, B. W., Jr., Feldman, M., & Quon, H. (2011). Transoral robotic surgery and human papillomavirus status: Oncologic results. *Head and Neck, 33*(4), 573–580.

Dean, N. R., Rosenthal, E. L., Carroll, W. R., Kostrzewa, J. P, Jones, V. L, Desmond, R. A, . . . Magnuson, J. S. (2010). Robotic-assisted surgery for primary or recurrent oropharyngeal carcinoma. *Archives of Otolaryngology-Head and Neck Surgery, 136*(4), 380–384.

de Arruda, F. F., Puri, D. R., Zhung, J., Narayana, A., Wolden, S., Hunt, M., . . . Lee, N. Y. (2006). Intensity-modulated radiation therapy for the treatment of oropharyngeal carcinoma: The Memorial Sloan-Kettering Cancer Center experience. *International Journal of Radiation Oncology Biology Physics, 64*(2), 363–373.

Forastiere, A. A., & Trotti, A. (1999). Radiotherapy and concurrent chemotherapy: A strategy that improves locoregional control and survival in oropharyngeal cancer. *Journal of the National Cancer Institute, 91*(24), 2065–2066.

Genital HPV Fact Sheet. *Sexually Transmitted Diseases (STDs)* 2011; http://www.cdc.gov/std/hpv/stdfact-hpv.htm .

Grant D. G., Salassa, J. R., Hinni, M. L., Pearson, B. W., & Perry, W. C. (2006). Carcinoma of the tongue base treated by transoral laser microsurgery, part one: Untreated tumors, a prospective analysis of oncologic and functional outcomes. *Laryngoscope, 116*(12), 2150–2155.

Hockstein, N. G., O'Malley, B. W., Jr., & Weinstein, G. S. (2006).Assessment of intraoperative safety in transoral robotic surgery. *Laryngoscope, 116*(2), 165–168.

Hockstein, N. G., Weinstein, G. S., & O'Malley, Jr., B. W. (2005). Maintenance of hemostasis in transoral robotic surgery. *ORL: Journal for Otorhinolaryngology and Its Related Specialties, 67*(4), 220–224.

Kumar, B., Cordell, K. G., Lee, J. S., Prince, M. E., Tran, H. H., Wolf, G. T., . . . Carey, T. E. (2007). Response to therapy and outcomes in oropharyngeal cancer are associated with biomarkers including human papillomavirus, epidermal growth factor receptor, gender, and smoking. *International Journal of Radiation Oncology Biology Physics, 69*(2 Suppl.), S109–S111.

Lawson, J. D., Otto, K., Chen, A., Shin, D. M., Davis, L., & Johnstone, P. A. (2006). Concurrent platinum-based chemotherapy and simultaneous modulated accelerated radiation therapy for locally advanced squamous cell carcinoma of the tongue base. *Head and Neck, 30*(3), 327–335.

O'Brien, C. J., Lee, K. K., Stern, H. S., Traynor, S. J., Bron, L, Tew, P. J., & Haghighi, K.S. (1998). Evaluation of 250 free-flap reconstructions after resection of tumours of the head and neck. *Austrailan and New Zealand Journal of Surgery, 68*(10), 698–701.

O'Malley, B. W., Jr., Quon, H., Leonhardt, F. D., Chalian, A. A., & Weinstein, G. S. (2010). Transoral robotic surgery for parapharyngeal space tumors. *ORL: Journal for Otorhinolaryngology and Its Related Specialties, 72*(6), 332–336.

O'Malley, B. W., Jr., Weinstein, G. S., & Hockstein, N. G. (2006). Transoral robotic surgery (TORS): Glottic microsurgery in a canine model. *Journal of Voice, 20*(2), 263–268.

O'Malley, B. W., Jr., Weinstein, G. S., Snyder, W., & Hockstein, N. G. (2006). Transoral robotic surgery (TORS) for base of tongue neoplasms. *Laryngoscope, 116*(8), 1465–1472.

Rusthoven, K. E., Raben, D., Ballonoff, A., Kane, M., Song, J. I., & Chen, C. (2008). Effect of radiation techniques in treatment of oropharynx cancer. *Laryngoscope, 118*(4), 635–639.

Sedaghat, A. R., Zhang, Z., Begum, S., Palermo, R., Best, S., Ulmer, K. M., . . . Pai, S. I. (2009). Prognostic significance of human papillomavirus in oropharyngeal squamous cell carcinomas. *Laryngoscope, 119*(8), 1542–1549.

Terrell, J. E., Ronis, D. L., Fowler, K. E., Bradford, C. R., Chepeha, D. B., Prince, M. E., . . . Duffy, S. A. (2004). Clinical predictors of quality of life in patients with head and neck cancer. *Archives of Otolaryngology-Head and Neck Surgery, 130*(4), 401–408.

Weinstein, G. S., O'Malley, B. W., Jr., Cohen, M. A., & Quon, H. (2010). Transoral robotic surgery for advanced oropharyngeal carcinoma. *Archives of Otolaryngology-Head and Neck Surgery, 136*(11), 1079–1085.

Weinstein, G. S., O'Malley, B. W., Jr., Snyder, W., & Hockstein, N. G. (2007). Transoral robotic surgery: Supraglottic partial laryngectomy. *Annals of Otology, Rhinology, and Laryngology, 116*(1), 19–23.

Weinstein, G. S., O'Malley, B. W., Jr., Snyder, W., Sherman, E., & Quon, H. (2007). Transoral robotic surgery: Radical tonsillectomy. *Archives of Otolaryngology Head and Neck Surgery, 133*(12), 1220–1226.

Yin Tsang, R. K., Ho, W. K., & Wei, W. I. (2011). Combined transnasal endoscopic and transoral robotic resection of recurrent nasopharyngeal carcinoma. *Head and Neck,* 2011 Mar 17. doi: 10.1002/hed.21731.

5

MEETING THE CHALLENGES OF RADIATION THERAPY

David S. Yoo, MD, PhD,
Mary Ann Downey Rubio, PA-C,
Gail Funk, RN, OCN,
Brandey Terruso, RD, CSO, LDN,
Linda Gilliard, MS, RD, CNSD,
David M. Brizel, MD

Nearly 50,000 people are diagnosed annually with an oral or other head and neck malignancy in the United States (Jemal, Siegel, Xu, & Ward, 2010). Approximately 90% are diagnosed as squamous cell carcinomas. Patients often present for medical attention after weeks or months of symptoms related to throat pain, ear pain, or difficulty with swallowing, with accompanying significant weight loss and nutritional compromise. Many times, patients also have a history of tobacco and/or alcohol use with pre-existing heart, lung, kidney, or liver conditions.

Management of these cancers therefore requires an integrated and multidisciplinary approach. During initial consultation, a patient may meet with a wide variety of specialists and providers, including otolaryngologists, radiation oncologists, medical oncologists, oral surgeons, radiologists, midlevel practitioners (physician assistants and nurse practitioners), nurses, dieticians, speech pathologists, social workers, counselors, and other patient advocates.

The objective with each patient is to come up with an individualized treatment plan that matches the goal of therapy (cure versus palliation) to the most appropriate treatment option(s), while maximizing the chances of the patient actually completing the prescribed therapy. For earlier stages of disease, single modality therapy with either surgery or radiation therapy alone may be sufficient for cure. More advanced stages of head and neck cancer typically require more intensive therapy, with some combination and sequence of surgery, radiotherapy, and systemic therapy. Of course, patients need to be healthy enough to tolerate these more aggressive regimens.

Radiation with concurrent chemotherapy are often used as first-line treatments to cure patients, with surgery reserved for persistent disease or recurrence, in order to preserve the underlying anatomic structures. However, there are times when the cancer has already destroyed enough of the normal tissue architecture that there is little functional organ left to preserve. In these situations, surgical removal of the tumor with reconstruction, rehabilitation, and postoperative radiation may provide cure with better overall quality of life.

For patients requiring radiation therapy, the fear and anxiety from their cancer diagnosis is often compounded by their fear and anxiety about radiation therapy. What is radiation therapy, and how does it work? At the most basic level, ionizing radiation kills cells by causing irreparable damage to DNA within the cancer cells and thus prevents further replication or cell division. Rapidly dividing cancer cells are more sensitive to the radiation than their normal nonmalignant counterparts, but these nonmalignant cells are also affected or damaged but in a sublethal way. The absorbed dose of radiation is expressed in units of gray (Gy), very similar to how drugs are discussed in terms of milligrams or teaspoons. The radiation oncologist's job is to focus the right dose of radiation to the appropriate areas, while respecting the tolerance of the surrounding normal tissues.

Radiotherapy is most commonly delivered via external beams such as photons (x-rays) and electrons generated by linear accelerators. High-energy photons can penetrate through the body to reach deep-seated tumors, whereas electrons are useful in treating tumors situated at more superficial depths. Some institutions utilize brachytherapy implants for head and neck cancer treatment. Brachytherapy involves the placement of radioactive sources in close proximity to a tumor to deliver the dose. Implants are usually placed in the operating room under anesthesia and are used in specialized circumstances. However, the use of more conformal radiation techniques such as intensity-modulated radiation therapy (IMRT) has further reduced the need to perform implants.

IMRT is now standard at virtually all academic radiation departments and most centers that treat large numbers of head and neck cancer patients. With more conventional two-dimensional (2-D) or three-dimensional (3-D) delivery techniques, the field sizes and shapes of each treatment portal are constant while the radiation beam is on. Some normal tissues can be shielded with custom blocks or a device called a multileaf collimator in the head of the treatment machine. By varying the actual amount of radiation transmitted at any point in time by these blocks and collimation devices, the intensity or dose of radiation can be modulated or "molded and shaped" to allow the tumor itself to receive the full dose. Therefore, as with former or 2-D treatment of tumors in the base of tongue or tonsil, the parotid glands would receive enough radiation to cause permanent damage and resultant xerostomia (dry mouth). With IMRT, the blocks and collimation in the treatment machine can be programmed to move during and within the radiation beam path to change its intensity in certain regions around the tumor itself. By treating this way, and from multiple different angles, the radiation dose distribution can be shaped to deliver full treatment to tumor targets while minimizing the dose around normal critical structures.

Increased sophistication in treatment planning and delivery requires precise and reproducible patient immobilization. During simulation, a custom head holder in the form of a mask is made for the patient by soaking a plastic mesh in warm water, stretching the now pliable material over the patient's face while he or she lies down in the treatment position, clamping the mesh frame to the planning table, and waiting while the plastic cools and hardens into shape. Breathing through the mask is not difficult, but claustrophobic or anxious patients may require a short-acting antianxiety medication in preparation for treatment sessions. Once the patient is immobilized in the treatment position, a CT scan is performed, with the resulting images used to plan the actual radiation therapy.

Curative courses and doses of radiation therapy typically last 6 to 7 weeks. The actual details with regard to the total dose prescribed, the total number of treatment fractions, the number of treatments per day, or which chemotherapy/molecular-targeted agents are used can differ depending on the stage of disease and the institution at which a patient is treated. A typical regimen for cure with radiation alone could consist of daily treatments, 5 days a week, for 35 treatments. Typically, a small dose of radiation (2 Gy) is given each day, with a total dose of 70 Gy for tumors that can be seen or felt on examination. For postoperative cases, 30 to 33 treatments are usually given, with doses in the 60 to 66-Gy range (Bernier et al., ,2005). However, other standard regimens treat patients twice a day with smaller individual fractions to a higher total dose, or 6 days a week to accelerate therapy (hyperfractionation), or a "concomitant boost" approach in which a patient starts with once a day treatments but ends up with two fractions per day during the last 2 weeks (Fu et al., 2000). These strategies, going to a higher dose, finishing treatment sooner, or giving an extra boost near the end, are designed to overcome cancer cells' mechanisms of resistance to radiation therapy.

For more advanced disease that is still curable, chemotherapy or molecular-targeted agents are given at the same time (concurrently) with radiation to improve treatment outcomes (Adelstein et al., 2002; Bonner et al., 2006; Brizel, Albers, et al., 1998). Some institutions give induction or so-called "up front" chemotherapy first for a few cycles, followed by concurrent chemotherapy and radiation. Whether this approach is better than standard chemoradiation alone is not yet known. Clinical trials are currently attempting to address this question. Examples of chemotherapy drugs and targeted agents used in head and neck cancer treatment regimens include cisplatin, 5-fluorouracil, paclitaxel, docetaxel, hydroxyurea, erlotinib (Tarceva), cetuximab (Erbitux), and bevacizumab (Avastin). Other drugs may be used routinely or in the setting of clinical trials depending on which institution is coordinating the treatment. As always, patient performance status, age, and co-existing medical conditions may influence the physician's treatment recommendations. In general, with more advanced disease, more intensive therapy is required to improve chances for cure, with the potential for more side effects and toxicity.

The development of side effects from radiation therapy depends on multiple factors, including the type and location of the primary tumor, the radiation technique used, the dose delivered, and the concurrent use of systemic agents. The responsibility of the multidisciplinary team is to monitor patients during therapy, anticipating problems and preparing patients for these toxicities—their usual time and mode of presentation, their severity, and their appropriate management to preserve the patient's functional status and prevent treatment breaks and delays. This is accomplished formally during the weekly on-treatment visit and whenever new problems arise.

Side effects are classified as either acute (early) or chronic (late). Acute toxicities occur during therapy and should begin to resolve within 2 to 3 months of radiotherapy completion. Chronic effects are those that typically arise once the acute side effects have subsided. Unfortunately, patients are at risk for the development of late effects for the remainder of their lives.

During the first weeks of therapy, patients commonly may experience mild to moderate fatigue. Some contributing factors, such as low blood counts or infection, are looked for and addressed with transfusions or antibiotics. Patients may also notice a change or loss of taste and decreased appetite. This is closely related to the changes in saliva discussed in greater detail below. Usually, taste returns to normal or near normal after treatment. Hair loss may occur in patches within the radiation treatment fields and is usually temporary but depends on the amount of radiation dose received.

Skin reactions may occur 3 to 4 weeks into therapy and range from skin redness (grade 1) to moist desquamation or shedding of the outer layers of the skin (grade 3). Meticulous skin care is important: cleaning with gentle soap and water, moisturizing with nonalcoholic lotion, and avoiding tight-fitting clothing that can rub and further irritate the area. Patients should not apply lotions in the 4 hours prior to treatment; however, they may be applied as needed after treatment. Skin reactions generally resolve within 2 to 3 weeks after completion of radiotherapy.

Patients receiving concurrent systemic or chemotherapy may also experience side effects specific to those agents. The chemotherapy drug, cisplatin, is used most often with radiation in head and neck cancers and can cause nausea and/or vomiting, decreased blood counts, hearing loss, and kidney problems. Patients receiving radiation alone occasionally can complain of nausea and vomiting, although many times, this is related to the thickened saliva and oral secretions that cause gagging and reflex coughing.

Thickened saliva and dry mouth (xerostomia) are major quality-of-life issues associated with head and neck radiation therapy. These can be temporary or permanent and vary in severity depending on the location of the tumor and the ability to spare salivary glands with radiation technique. Sometimes, tumors are very close to or even touch the parotid glands, making sparing of these structures very difficult in terms of sparing salivary gland tissue. In these situations, killing the tumor takes priority over sparing the glands.

A number of over-the-counter artificial saliva substitutes are available that may help with dry mouth. A solution of 1:3 parts peroxide to water used as a gargle can help break up the mucus and make it easier to clear. Additionally, guaifenesin, an over-the-counter mucolytic or mucus thinning agent, can thin the secretions and make them more manageable. This comes in liquid and pill form but must be taken with increased fluids to be effective. If dry mouth persists and does not respond to artificial saliva products, there are medications that can be prescribed, including pilocarpine (Salagen) and cevimeline (Evoxac). They are beneficial in 30 to 50% of patients but have side effects and cannot be taken if the patient has certain heart problems, emphysema, or glaucoma. Amifostine (Ethyol), a drug that can be administered intravenously or subcutaneously prior to each daily dose of radiation, may reduce the incidence and severity of xerostomia and was approved by the FDA for use in the setting of once-daily postoperative radiation therapy (Brizel, Wasserman, et al., 2000). Whether amifostine has similar benefits in the context of definitive radiation therapy or with concurrent chemotherapy or for the prevention of other treatment-related complications has not been established. Moreover, the use of IMRT to spare the salivary glands has also significantly reduced the incidence of long-term xerostomia after treatment.

Alterations in the properties of saliva following radiation treatment may predispose patients to oral fungal infections and tooth decay. It is of utmost importance that all patients with head and neck cancer planning to undergo radiation therapy have a thorough dental evaluation prior to the start of treatments, with frequent follow-up care and emphasis on preventive dental care. Following completion of radiation, routine dental evaluation and cleaning should be performed every 3 to 4 months until salivary function has returned to normal.

Mouth pain, throat pain, or painful swallowing is variable in onset and highly dependent on type and location of tumor as well as radiation technique. Generally, symptoms become noticeable within 2 weeks of starting radiotherapy. These signs and symptoms are collectively referred to as mucositis. They are severe in at least 50% of patients who receive radiation with concurrent chemotherapy. Local anesthetics such as over-the-counter Sucrets, Chloroseptic, or prescription viscous lidocaine are used initially, followed by anti-inflammatory drugs. Most patients eventually require both short-acting and long-acting narcotic pain medications. Often, a combination of several different drugs is required to adequately control pain.

The goal is to keep the pain below a 3 on the 0 to 10 pain scale (10 being "unbearable") so patients are able to eat and drink in a manner that allows maintenance of hydration and caloric intake. Pain control is important, as changes in taste alteration, fatigue, nausea, and saliva changes already conspire to take away the normal appetite and desire of patients to eat. Some institutions will prophylactically put percutaneous feeding tubes ("G-tube" or "PEG tube") in all head and neck cancer patients to prevent weight loss (Beer et al., 2005; Nguyen et al., 2006). Others believe in a more proactive and reactive approach, with percutaneous tubes reserved for patients who have exhausted aggressive medical and multidisciplinary supportive management, including temporary nasogastric feeding tubes (Clavel et al., 2011; Corry et al., 2008; Lawson et al., 2009).

Adequate nutrition before, during, and after radiotherapy is crucial to the completion of treatment and to proper healing after radiation is completed (Paccagnella et al., 2010). Increasing the probability of timely and successful treatment completion can improve the chances for overall survival. Early dietary intervention with a registered dietitian (RD) has been demonstrated to help with recovery from treatment side effects and improve quality of life (Colasanto et al., 2005; Dawson et al., 2001; Larsson et al., 2005; Munshi et al., 2003). One randomized prospective clinical trial has also shown that nutritional intervention could improve the quality of life in head and neck cancer patients (Ravasco et al., 2005). Intensive professional nutritional support by an RD who has Board Certification in Oncology Nutrition (CSO) is suggested.

A medical nutrition therapy (MNT) plan is strongly advised, with consultation prior to or early on in treatment, with weekly monitoring during therapy and subsequent post-therapy follow-up monthly for at least one year (American Dietetic Aassociation, 2010). If significant weight loss has occurred prior to diagnosis, it is important that dietary interventions be implemented to discourage further weight loss. In patients who are already nutritionally compromised or major nutritional problems are anticipated, a feeding tube should be considered prior to beginning radiation therapy. Other causes of weight loss should be investigated. If lower intake is due to a loss of appetite, then education on making foods calorically dense in small quantities and eating more frequently throughout the day will encourage weight maintenance. If chewing and swallowing certain textures has become difficult, then eating softer foods and liquids that are dense with calories is the goal. Nutritional drinks such as Ensure Plus, Boost Plus, or Carnation Instant Breakfast Plus are beneficial supplements to the diet. Generic nutritional supplements, which are comparable to the nutritional supplements listed above, are also suggested due to being lower in cost with similar nutritional composition of calories and grams of protein per serving.

If there has been no weight loss prior to radiotherapy, then continuing to maintain weight throughout treatment is the goal. Monitoring weight closely by using the same scale at the same time of day, several days per week will help to avoid unexpected rapid weight loss. Adding an appropriate snack or supplement or making foods calorically dense are necessary dietary changes that should be made if weight loss occurs at any point during treatment. If weight maintenance is not possible by eating and drinking, placement of feeding tubes (either nasogastric or percutaneous) should be considered.

Late effects from radiation therapy that can develop over time include permanent dry mouth, dental decay, osteoradionecrosis (death of bone tissue), soft tissue necrosis, swallowing difficulties with permanent feeding tube dependence, carotid artery stenosis (narrowing), hypothyroidism, brachial plexus injury, scarring or edema of structures in the treatment field, and, rarely, the risk of radiation-induced second malignancy. Any of these outcomes should be discussed with a radiation oncologist.

In conclusion, radiation therapy is the standard nonsurgical treatment for head and neck cancers. Concurrent chemotherapy and radiation therapy is the standard of care for locally advanced disease when the tumor is unresectable or surgical options carry significant functional morbidity or side effects. Postoperative radiation may also be delivered for patients deemed at high risk of recurrence with surgery alone. Treatment demands a knowledgeable team, expert in therapy delivery. Ongoing improvements in technology have increased the chances of cure with lesser long-term side effects. However, compliance and follow-up is paramount to the likelihood of success and the overall quality of life for survivors. In that context, the broader multidisciplinary team also plays a crucial role through the skilled management of the various toxicities that occur during and after treatment.

References

Adelstein, D. J., Saxton, J. P., Lavertu, P., Rybicki, L. A., Esclamado, R. M., Wood, B. G., . . . Carroll, M. A. (2002). Maximizing local control and organ preservation in stage IV squamous cell head and neck cancer With hyperfractionated radiation and concurrent chemotherapy. *Journal of Clinical Oncology: Official Journal of the American Society of Clinical Oncology, 20*(5), 1405–1410.

American Dietetic Association. (2010). Oncology toolkit, the Gold standard companion to ADA's evidence-based nutrition practice guideline. *MNT summary page for oncology nutrition. Head and neck cancer* (pp. 1–10). Chicago, IL: Author.

Beer, K. T., Krause, K. B., Zuercher, T., & Stanga, Z. (2005). Early percutaneous endoscopic gastrostomy insertion maintains nutritional state in patients with aerodigestive tract cancer. *Nutrition and Cancer, 52*(1), 29–34.

Bernier, J., Cooper, J. S., Pajak, T. F., van Glabbeke, M., Bourhis, J., Forastiere, A., . . . Lefèbvre, J. L. (2005). Defining risk levels in locally advanced head and neck cancers: A comparative analysis of concurrent postoperative radiation plus chemotherapy trials of the EORTC (#22931) and RTOG (# 9501). *Head and Neck, 27*(10), 843–850.

Bonner, J. A., Harari, P. M., Giralt, J., Azarnia, N., Shin, D. M., Cohen, R. B., . . . Jones, C. U. (2006). Radiotherapy plus cetuximab for squamous-cell carcinoma of the head and neck. *New England Journal of Medicine, 354*(6), 567–578.

Brizel, D. M., Albers, M. E., Fisher, S. R., Scher, R. L., Richtsmeier, W. J., Vera Hars, M.S., . . . Prosnitz, L. R. (1998). Hyperfractionated irradiation with or without concurrent chemotherapy for locally advanced head and neck cancer. *New England Journal of Medicine, 338*(25), 1798–1804.

Brizel, D. M., Wasserman, T. H., Henke, M., Strnad, V., Rudat, V., Monnier, A., . . . Sauer, R. (2000). Phase III randomized trial of amifostine as a radioprotector in head and neck cancer. *Journal of Clinical Oncology: Official Journal of the American Society of Clinical Oncology, 18*(19), 3339–3345.

Clavel, S., Fortin, B., Després, P., Donath, D., Soulières, D., Khaouam, N., . . . Nguyen-Tan, P. F. (2011). Enteral feeding during chemoradiotherapy for advanced head-and-neck cancer: A single-institution experience using a reactive approach. *International Journal of Radiation Oncology, Biology, Physics, 79*(3), 763–769.

Colasanto, J. M., Prasad, P., Nash, M. A., Decker, R. H., & Wilson, L. D. (2005). Nutritional support of patients undergoing radiation therapy for head and neck cancer. *Oncology, 19*(3), 371–379; discussion 380–372, 387.

Corry, J., Poon, W., McPhee, N., Milner, A. D., Cruickshank, D., Porceddu, S. V., . . . Peters, L. J. (2008). Randomized study of percutaneous endoscopic gastrostomy versus nasogastric tubes for enteral feeding in head and neck cancer patients treated with (chemo)radiation. *Journal of Medical Imaging and Radiation Oncology, 52*(5), 503–510.

Dawson, E. R., Morley, S. E., Robertson, A. G., & Soutar, D. S. (2001). Increasing dietary supervision can reduce weight loss in oral cancer patients. *Nutrition and Cancer, 41*(1–2), 70–74.

Fu, K. K., Pajak, T. F., Trotti, A., Jones, C. U., Spencer, S. A., Phillips, T. L., . . . Ang, K. K. (2000). A Radiation Therapy Oncology Group (RTOG) phase III randomized study to compare hyperfractionation and two variants of accelerated fractionation to standard fractionation radiotherapy for head and neck squamous cell carcinomas: First report of

RTOG 9003. *International Journal of Radiation Oncology, Biology, Physics, 48*(1), 7–16.

Jemal, A., Siegel, R., Xu, J., & Ward, E. (2010). Cancer statistics, 2010. *CA: A Cancer Journal for Clinicians, 60*(5), 277–300.

Larsson, M., Hedelin, B., Johansson, I., & Athlin, E. (2005). Eating problems and weight loss for patients with head and neck cancer: A chart review from diagnosis until one year after treatment. *Cancer Nursing, 28*(6), 425–435.

Lawson, J. D., Gaultney, J., Saba, N., Grist, W., Davis, L., & Johnstone, P. A. (2009). Percutaneous feeding tubes in patients with head and neck cancer: Rethinking prophylactic placement for patients undergoing chemoradiation. *American Journal of Otolaryngology, 30*(4), 244–249.

Munshi, A., Pandey, M. B., Durga, T., Pandey, K. C., Bahadur, S., & Mohanti, B. K. (2003). Weight loss during radiotherapy for head and neck malignancies: What factors impact it? *Nutrition and Cancer, 47*(2), 136–140.

Nguyen, N. P., North, D., Smith, H. J., Dutta, S., Alfieri, A., Karlsson, U., . . . Sallah, S. (2006). Safety and effectiveness of prophylactic gastrostomy tubes for head and neck cancer patients undergoing chemoradiation. *Surgical Oncology, 15*(4), 199–203.

Paccagnella, A., Morello, M., Da Mosto, M. C., Baruffi, C., Marcon, M. L., Gava, A., . . . Marchiori, C. (2010). Early nutritional intervention improves treatment tolerance and outcomes in head and neck cancer patients undergoing concurrent chemoradiotherapy. *Supportive Care in Cancer: Official Journal of the Multinational Association of Supportive Care in Cancer, 18*(7), 837–845.

Ravasco, P., Monteiro-Grillo, I., Marques Vidal, P., & Camilo, M. E. (2005). Impact of nutrition on outcome: A prospective randomized controlled trial in patients with head and neck cancer undergoing radiotherapy. *Head and Neck, 27*(8), 659–668.

6

MEETING THE CHALLENGES OF CHEMOTHERAPY IN THE TREATMENT OF ORAL AND HEAD AND NECK CANCER

Su Hsien Lim, MD, Shrujal Baxi, MD, MPH,
Matthew Fury, MD, PhD
David G. Pfister, MD

Treating Head and Neck Squamous Cell Carcinoma with Chemotherapy

Historically, surgery and radiation therapy have been the cornerstones of treatment for head and neck squamous cell cancers (HNSCC), especially when the disease is limited to being located above the collarbones and cure is possible. Chemotherapy alone rarely leads to a cure for these tumors and has formerly been used mainly for patients in whom disease has recurred or spread to a distant site, in hopes of prolonging survival and relieving symptoms. However, the results of clinical trials over the past 20 years have provided the basis for a much greater role for chemotherapy and clarified both when and how to use drug therapy in conjunction with radiation and surgery to improve disease control.

What Is Chemotherapy and Why Is It Given?

Cancer develops when cells in a part of the body begin to grow in an abnormal and uncontrolled manner. Chemotherapy involves use of drug treatment to either control the multiplication of or kill these abnormal cancer cells, thus causing tumors to shrink and prevent their spread. When it is given along with other treatments, such as radiation, chemotherapy can also improve the effectiveness of those treatments.

There are many different types of chemotherapy drugs that work by interfering with various parts of a cancer cell's internal structure and function or the process of cell division or duplication. Newer "targeted" agents, including monoclonal antibodies (proteins designed to target a specific site on the cancer cell) and hormonal treatments work by affecting very specific metabolic processes.

How and When Is Chemotherapy Used in the Treatment of Head and Neck Cancer?

There are several different indications for the use of chemotherapy in the treatment of HNSCC.

Treatment of Locally or Regionally Advanced Disease

Locoregionally advanced disease is defined as the presence of a large primary tumor or tumors with spread to neck lymph nodes, but have not spread beyond the head and neck region. These cancers are treated with the intention of cure, but the prognosis is worse than in patients with less advanced disease. Historically, the treatment approach for these advanced cancers has depended on whether surgery was possible. When operable, patients generally underwent surgery followed by postoperative radiation therapy. However, surgery in this setting may lead to altered facial appearance and difficulties with key functions such as speaking, chewing, and swallowing despite advances in surgical techniques and reconstruction. Larger tumors that could not be surgically removed were treated with radiation alone with disappointing cure rates.

In patients with locoregionally advanced disease, chemotherapy can be used with surgery and/or radiation in three main ways: concurrently (at the same time) with radiation, as adjuvant therapy (after surgery or radiation), or as induction/neoadjuvant therapy (before other treatment).

■ *Concurrent chemoradiation*, or chemotherapy given at the same time as radiation therapy, is more effective than radiation alone to control tumors that cannot be surgically removed (Adelstein et al., 2003; Brizel et al., 1998; Fountzilas et al., 2004; Pignon et al., 2000; Pignon et al., 2009), including advanced nasopharyngeal carcinoma (Al-Sarraf et al., 1998), advanced oropharyngeal cancer (Calais et al., 1999), and in the adjuvant setting after surgery in patients with disease at high risk for relapse as discussed next (Bernier et al., 2004; Cooper et al., 2004). It also achieves a better rate of organ preservation, such as preservation of the larynx, than radiotherapy alone (Forastiere et al., 2006), thus offering patients the option of avoiding surgery without compromise in cure rates.

■ *Adjuvant therapy*, or therapy given after primary treatment, is used when patients are found at surgery to have high-risk pathologic features (that is, features in their tumors worrisome for more aggressive behavior and is associated with a greater likelihood of recurrence). The addition of adjuvant therapy is intended to decrease the risk of relapse. Historically, adjuvant treatment has been in association with radiation therapy alone; chemotherapy alone has not been shown to improve survival. However, recent studies have found that the addition of cisplatin chemotherapy concurrently with radiation therapy significantly improves disease control above the collarbones in patients at a higher risk of relapse (Bernier et al., 2004; Cooper et al., 2004). On a collective analysis of both studies, two pathological features were particularly associated with benefit from the incorporation of chemotherapy: the presence of cancer cells at the surgical margins (positive margins), or the extension of tumor cells outside of lymph nodes into the surrounding tissue (extracapsular spread or extension) (Bernier et al., 2005).

■ *Neoadjuvant therapy*, or chemotherapy given prior to definitive therapy with either surgery and/or radiation to the primary site and neck, was the focus of several randomized clinical trials during the 1980s and 1990s. Although tumors can demonstrate significant shrinkage with related palliation of symptoms, and the incidence of distant metastases may decrease with the use of induction chemotherapy, a collective analysis of these studies (meta-analysis) failed to demonstrate a convincing benefit to overall survival with the addition of chemotherapy in this manner (Pignon et al., 2000; Pignon et al., 2009).

However, there is renewed interest in induction/neoadjuvant therapy for two reasons. First, more effective treatment for locoregional disease has resulted in better control of tumors above the collarbones, such that the development of metastatic disease to other sites in the body has become a more common type of treatment failure. Induction chemotherapy is one way to potentially decrease the rate of these distant metastases. Second, newer triplet combination chemotherapy regimens (either docetaxel or paclitaxel, combined with cisplatin and 5-fluororuacil) appear more effective than the historically used doublet of cisplatin and 5-fluorouracil alone (Hitt et al., 2005; Posner et al., 2007; Vermorken et al., 2007). Studies comparing concurrent chemoradiation alone to induction triplet chemotherapy followed by chemoradiation are in progress to determine whether the latter approach improves survival compared with the former one and to what extent the toxicity of treatment is also increased.

Treatment of Recurrent or Metastatic Disease

Locoregional recurrence of HNSCC refers to disease that has come back in the head and neck area but has not spread anywhere else in the body. In this case, surgery and/or radiation may be used with the intent of cure and is successful to this end in selected patients. If neither surgery nor radiation is possible for new locoregional relapse, or if the cancer has spread to other body regions, the prognosis is much worse. Selected patients may benefit from surgical removal of a distant site of disease, particularly if limited to the lungs, but chemotherapy alone is more commonly used in this situation. The goals of treatment are prolongation of life, decrease in symptoms, and improvement in quality of life. These patients, on average, live less than a year when treated with available standard anticancer drugs; therefore, clinical trials evaluating promising new agents are often an excellent option and deserve consideration.

First-line therapy in the recurrent or metastatic setting often consists of a platinum-based doublet. Commonly used examples include cisplatin combined with other drugs active in HNSCC such as paclitaxel or 5-fluorouracil. The rates of major tumor shrinkage with these treatments are approximately 30 to 40%, but the duration generally is measured in weeks to months, and a significant survival advantage compared with treatment with single drugs that have lower response rates but also lower side effects is not well established (Cohen, Lingen, & Vokes, 2004). Second-line therapies typically employ a single agent, offer lower response rates, and have a disappointing impact with regard to prolonging survival (Leon et al., 2005).

What Types of Chemotherapy Are Being Used Today?

Active classic chemotherapeutic agents for HNSCC include, but are not limited to, methotrexate, cisplatin, carboplatin, 5-fluorouracil, paclitaxel, docetaxel, gemcitabine (for nasopharynx cancer), and bleomycin. Each of these drugs works differently to control the growth, multiplication, and survival of cancer cells. The anticipated rates of major tumor shrinkage in the relapsed or metastatic disease setting when a single drug is used are approximately 10 to 20%; using a combination of drugs doubles the major response rates. The tumor shrinkage rates further improve when drugs are used as the initial (induction/neoadjuvant) treatment prior to surgery or radiation.

Given the somewhat disappointing effectiveness of current chemotherapy regimens for recurrent or metastatic HNSCC, there is much ongoing research to identify new and better drugs. There is particular interest in agents that look to exploit newly identified molecular targets in cancer cells and thus offer the hope for treatment that is more specific to the tumor and less toxic to the noncancerous normal tissue. Cetuximab is an example of such a drug. Cetuximab is a monoclonal antibody that targets the epidermal growth factor receptor (EGFR), a structure expressed on the surface of most HNSCC cells involved in the growth and spread of disease. Cetuximab was approved by the Food and Drug Administration in 2006 for use in the primary treatment of HNSCC concurrently with radiation as well as for recurrent or metastatic disease that no longer responds to cisplatin. Furthermore, data from a recent study indicate that it provides added anticancer effect and improvement in survival when combined with a platinum-based doublet in the first-line setting compared to treatment with a platinum-based doublet alone (Vermorken et al., 2008).

Another example of an area of interest for targeted cancer treatment is the development of drugs that interfere with the process of angiogenesis (the creation of blood vessels that feed the tumor). Angiogenesis is promoted by vascular endothelial growth factor (VEGF). Bevacizumab is an example of an anti-angiogenesis therapy, being an antibody that binds to VEGF and prevents it from inducing blood vessel growth into tumors. Unlike cetuximab, bevacizumab is not currently approved by the Food and Drug Administration for the treatment of HNSCC. Clinical trials evaluating the potential role of bevacizumab in the treatment of SCHNC are currently ongoing.

How Are Chemotherapy Drugs Given?

Most commonly, chemotherapy is delivered directly into the bloodstream through an intravenous catheter. The drug typically is diluted in intravenous fluid prior to administration. Increasingly, chemotherapy is becoming available in oral form as a pill or capsule.

Although a single chemotherapy drug can be given, different drugs are frequently given in combination. The rationale for this strategy is to reduce the chance that the cancer cells will be resistant or will develop resistance to the drugs administered. However, when multiple drugs are given, the side effects are usually greater. The intent of treatment (curative versus palliative), anticipated efficacy, expected side effects, and patient tolerance are all considered when selecting a chemotherapy program.

Chemotherapy is frequently administered in cycles. The length of the cycle varies depending on the drug and the regimen.

These cycle lengths have been previously determined based on the way the body metabolizes the drugs and prior studies. Depending on the agent or drug combination, dosing may range from daily administration to treatment every 3 to 4 weeks, with time off given in between cycles.

The overall duration of a course of chemotherapy will vary. Sometimes it is set, for example, with induction/neoadjuvant, concurrent, or adjuvant therapy, when a specified number of therapy cycles are planned. Other times, such as when the principal intent of treatment is not to cure but rather to decrease symptoms, it is given until maximum response occurs or limiting side effects develop, which typically happens within 4 to 6 months. Response to chemotherapy is generally assessed by physical exam or imaging approximately every 2 months. If tumor growth continues, a change in therapy is indicated.

What Are the Side Effects of Chemotherapy and What Can Be Done to Minimize and Alleviate Them?

Chemotherapy targets rapidly growing or dividing cells. This includes not only the cancers cells but also normal cells such as hair follicles, the cells lining the gastrointestinal tract, reproductive cells (sperm), and blood-forming cells. Side effects from chemotherapy are caused by the disruption of the proper function of these cells. Patients may experience alopecia (hair loss), diarrhea, nausea, mouth sores, decreased fertility, increased risk of infection, anemia, bleeding, and generalized fatigue and weakness.

Specific drugs have their own side effects in addition to the more general side effects of chemotherapy. Examples may include nerve effects manifested as numbness and tingling of the hands and feet, hearing loss and ringing in the ears, decline in kidney function, decline in the heart's function, damage to the liver, rash, and derangements in the blood's ability to clot.

In addition, there is the risk of a hypersensitivity or allergic reaction to some chemotherapy regimens. Symptoms of hypersensitivity range from mild effects such as rash to rare but life-threatening ones such as shock. For chemotherapy drugs that are prone to cause hypersensitivity, pretreatment with certain medications such as antihistamines and steroids is employed. If a reaction nonetheless occurs, additional medication will be administered or use of that particular chemotherapy may need to be discontinued.

The extent of side effects experienced by any one patient varies. Several different drugs and approaches can be used to minimize and alleviate the side effects. Nausea and vomiting can be minimized with the use of drugs before or after treatment. Examples include dexamethasone (a steroid); aprepitant; and 5-HT3 receptor antagonists such as palonosetron, ondansetron, dolasetron, granisetron, and alosetron. Other antinausea medicines may be given as needed, such as metoclopramide, prochlorperazine, and lorazepam.

The blood count must be monitored very closely in patients undergoing chemotherapy, and if the number of cells is too low, chemotherapy may be postponed until the blood count improves. Colony-stimulating agents are proteins that the body produces to induce production of certain blood components that can now be manufactured for external administration. Erythropoetin or darbepoetin may be administered if the red blood cell count is low and the patient is experiencing fatigue, weakness, or shortness of breath, but it is not recommended concurrently during radiation treatment, because the effectiveness of therapy may be adversely affected (Henke et al., 2003) In addition it is not recommended during bone marrow-suppressive therapy when administered with curative intent. Granulocyte colony-stimulating factor (GCSF) (e.g., filgrastim) may be administered for a low white blood cell count or as a preventive measure if the course of chemotherapy to be given is known to significantly suppress the white blood cell count; however, its use, concurrent with active radiation therapy is less well understood and generally is avoided in this setting.

Other drugs are given to minimize the side effects of radiation treatment. Amifostine is sometimes given during treatment to decrease the incidence of acute and chronic dry mouth (Brizel et al., 2000) but can be associated with side effects of its own (e.g., nausea and low blood pressure). Pilocarpine and cevimeline have been found to improve saliva production and symptoms of dry mouth as well (Chambers et al., 2007; Johnson et al., 1993).

To minimize toxicity to the kidneys from certain chemotherapy drugs, adequate fluid intake is ensured by infusion of saline prior to, during, and after administration of chemotherapy. Furthermore, it is confirmed prior to the start of treatment that the patient has a good urine output to make sure the drug will be cleared by the kidneys. Kidney function is also monitored, and if the kidney demonstrates disturbances in its ability to regulate and retain the electrolytes (minerals such as potassium and magnesium) that the body requires, supplementation of particular electrolytes may be necessary. If there is persistent deterioration in kidney function, the offending chemotherapeutic drug may need to be decreased or stopped.

Damage to the nerves resulting in neuropathy is associated with certain chemotherapies. Vitamin supplementation may help (e.g., vitamin B12). Also, certain medications may decrease the severity of symptoms (e.g., amitriptyline and pregabalin). However, if the neuropathy becomes debilitating, the chemotherapy drug is usually stopped.

Certain drugs may cause inflammation of the liver. Patients with significant liver involvement by the cancer may be more vulnerable to this side effect because they often have a less normally functioning liver when they start treatment, although this is uncommon in head and neck cancers. Regular blood tests are performed to check on the function of the liver. Intake of substances potentially toxic to the liver, such as acetaminophen and alcohol, should be minimized and monitored during treatment.

Chemotherapy may result in temporary or permanent sterility (inability to have children). In men, this is caused by a decline or cessation in sperm production; in women, this is due to changes in the menstrual cycle resulting in irregular or infrequent menses.

Menopause may occur in some women who are perimeno-pausal. In younger women the menstrual cycle often resumes and fertility returns. Many men choose to bank their sperm in anticipation of receiving chemotherapy; assisted reproductive technologies (e.g., egg banking) are available for women. Because of concerns regarding the teratogenic effects of chemotherapy drugs (causing malformations and defects to the fetus), precautions to prevent pregnancy should be taken throughout treatment with these agents.

Targeted therapies have well-known side effects and toxicities, too. With more widespread use of these agents, there is also a greater understanding about the management of these adverse effects (Bernier et al., 2008) For example, treatment with cetuximab results in an acneiform rash in most patients. This rash resolves after treatment, and is treated with topical and/ or systemic measures depending on its severity. Some patients can also have severe allergic reactions. Targeting of VEGF by bevacizumab may result in severe bleeding and impaired wound healing, blood clots, and esophageal perforation. Elevated blood pressure and protein in the urine are common but typically simple to control, and they subside once treatment is complete.

In summary, the role of chemotherapy in the treatment of HNSCC has evolved considerably over the past 20 years. The changes have been particularly dramatic among patients with locally or regionally advanced disease, in which chemotherapy figures prominently in the management of unresectable disease, nasopharynx cancer, oropharynx cancer, organ preservation programs, and the poor risk adjuvant setting. Although treatment with chemotherapy certainly carries risks and side effects, there are significant benefits from its use regarding disease control. Close monitoring and management by the treating oncologist minimizes the impact of treatment side effects.

The continued development of new drugs in the fight against HNSCC is critical. Well-done clinical trials are a fundamental part of this process and greatly assist in determining how and when to optimally use chemotherapy to improve disease control outcomes. These studies are often an excellent treatment option for patients and deserve support and participation whenever possible.

References

Adelstein, D. J., Li, Y., Adams, G. L.,Wagner, H., Jr., Kish, J. A., Ensley, J. F., . . . Forastiere, A. A. (2003). An intergroup phase III comparison of standard radiation therapy and two schedules of concurrent chemoradiotherapy in patients with unresectable squamous cell head and neck cancer. *Journal of Clinical Oncology, 21,* 92–98.

Al-Sarraf, M., LeBlanc, M., Giri, P. G., Fu, K. K., Cooper, J., Vuong, T., . . . Ensley, J. F. (1998). Chemoradiotherapy versus radiotherapy in patients with advanced nasopharyngeal cancer: Phase III randomized intergroup study 0099. *Journal of Clinical Oncology, 16,* 1310–1317.

Bernier, J., Bonner J., Vermorken, J. B., Bensadoun, R. J. Dumme, R., Giralt, J., . . . Ang, K. K. (2008). Consensus guidelines for the management of radiation dermatitis and coexisting acne-like rash in patients receiving radiotherapy plus EGFR inhibitors for the treatment of squamous cell carcinoma of the head and neck. *Annals of Oncology, 19,* 142–149

Bernier, J., Cooper, J. S., Pajak,T. F., van Glabbeke, M., Bourhis, J., Forastiere, A. A., . . . Lefèbvre, J. L. (2005). Defining risk levels in locally advanced head and neck cancers: A comparative analysis of concurrent postoperative radiation plus chemotherapy trials of the EORTC (#22931) and RTOG (#9501). *Head and Neck, 27,* 843–850.

Bernier, J., Domenge, C., Ozsahin, M., Matuszewska, K., Lefebvre, J. L., Greiner, R. H., . . . van Glabbeke, M. (2004). Postoperative irradiation with or without concomitant chemotherapy for locally advanced head and neck cancer. *New England Journal of Medicine, 350,* 1945–1952.

Brizel, D. M., Albers, M. E., Fisher, S. R., Scher, R. L., Richtsmeier, W. J., Hars, V., . . . Prosnitz, L. R. (1998). Hyperfractionated irradiation with or without concurrent chemotherapy for locally advanced head and neck cancer. *New England Journal of Medicine, 338,* 1798–1804.

Brizel, D. M., Wasserman, T. H., Henke, M., Strnad, V., Rudat, V., Monnier, A., . . . Sauer, R. (2000). Phase III randomized trial of amifostine as a radioprotector in head and neck cancer. *Journal of Clinical Oncology, 18*(24), 4110–4111.

Calais, G., Alfonsi, M., Bardet, E., Sire, C., Germain, T., Bergerot, P., . . . Bertrand, P. (1999). Randomized trial of radiation therapy versus concomitant chemotherapy and radiation therapy for advanced-stage oropharynx carcinoma. *Journal of the National Cancer Institute, 91,* 2081–2086.

Chambers, M. S., Posner, M., Jones, C. U., Biel, M. A., Hodge, K. M., Vitti, R., . . . Weber, R. S. (2007). Cevimeline for the treatment of post-irradiation xerostomia in patients with head and neck cancer. *International Journal of Radiation Oncology, Biology, Physics, 68*(4), 1102–1109.

Cohen, E. E., Lingen, M. W., & Vokes, E. E. (2004). The expanding role of systemic therapy in head and neck cancer. *Journal of Clinical Oncology, 22,* 1743–1752.

Cooper, J. S., Pajak, T. F., Forastiere, A. A., Jacobs, J., Campbell, B. H., Saxman, S. B., . . . Fu, K. K.(2004). Postoperative concurrent radiotherapy and chemotherapy for high-risk squamous-cell carcinoma of the head and neck. *New England Journal of Medicine, 350,* 1937–1944.

Forastiere, A. A., Maor, M., Weber, R., Pajak, T., Glisson, B., Trotti, A., . . . Cooper, J. (2006). Long-term results of intergroup RTOG 91-11: A phase III trial to preserve the larynx—Induction cisplatin/5FU and radiation therapy versus concurrent cisplatin and radiation therapy versus radiation therapy. *Journal of Clinical Oncology, 24,* Abstract 5517.

Fountzilas, G., Ciuleanu, E., Dafni, U., Plataniotis, G., Kalogera-Fountzila, A., Samantas, E., . . . Ghilezan, N.. (2004). Concomitant radiochemotherapy vs radiotherapy alone in patients with head and neck cancer: A Hellenic Cooperative Oncology Group phase III study. *Medical Oncology, 21,* 95–107.

Henke, M., Laszig, R., Rube, C., Schafer, U., Haase, K. D., Schilcher, B., . . . Frommhold, H. (2003). Erythropoietin to treat head and neck cancer patients with anemia undergoing radiotherapy: Randomized, double-blind, placebo controlled trial. *Lancet, 362*(9392), 1255–1260.

Hitt, R., Lopez-Pousa, A., Martinez-Trufero, J., Escrig, V., Carles, J., Rizo, A., . . . Cortés-Funes, H. (2005). Phase III study comparing cisplatin plus fluorouracil to paclitaxel, cisplatin, and fluorouracil induction chemotherapy followed by chemoradiotherapy in locally advanced head and neck cancer. *Journal of Clinical Oncology, 23,* 8636–8645.

Johnson, J. T., Ferretti, G. A., Nethery, W. J., Valdez, I. H., Fox, P. C., Ng, D., . . . Gallagher, S. (1993). Oral pilocarpine for post-irradiation xerostomia in patients with head and neck cancer. *New England Journal of Medicine, 329,* 390–395.

Leon, X., Hitt, R., Constenla, M., Rocca, A., Stupp, R., Kovacs, A. F., . . . Bourhis, J.(2005). A retrospective analysis of the outcome of patients with recurrent and/or metastatic squamous cell carcinoma of the head and neck refractory to a platinum-based chemotherapy. *Clinical Oncology (Royal College of Radiologists), 17,* 418–424.

Pignon, J. P., Bourhis, J., Domenge, C., & Designe, L. (2000). Chemotherapy added to locoregional treatment for head and neck squamous-cell carcinoma: Three meta-analyses of updated individual data. MACH-NC Collaborative Group. Meta-analysis of chemotherapy on head and neck cancer. *Lancet, 355,* 949–955.

Pignon, J. P., le Maitre, A., Maillard, E., Bourhis, J., & MACH-NC Collaborative Group. (2009). Meta-analysis of chemotherapy in head and neck cancer (MACH-NC): An update on 93 randomised trials and 17,346 patients. *Radiotherapy and Oncology, 92,* 4–14.

Posner, M. R., Hershock, D. M., Blajman, C. R., Mickiewicz, E.,Winquist, E., Gorbounova, E., . . .TAX 324 Study Group. (2007). Cisplatin and fluorouracil alone or with docetaxel in head and neck cancer. *New England Journal of Medicine, 357,* 1705–1715.

Vermorken, J. B., Mesia, R., Rivera, F., Remenar, E., Kawecki, A, Rottey, S., . . . Hitt, R. (2008). Platinum-based chemotherapy plus cetuximab in head and neck cancer. *New England Journal of Medicine, 359,* 1116–1127.

Vermorken, J. B., Remenar, E., van Herpen, C., Gorlia, T., Mesia, R., Degardin, M., . . . (2007). Cisplatin, fluorouracil, and docetaxel in unresectable head and neck cancer. *New England Journal of Medicine, 357,* 1695–1704.

7

MEETING THE CHALLENGES OF GOOD ORAL CARE IN THE MANAGEMENT OF HEAD AND NECK CANCER

James J. Sciubba, DMD, PhD

The management of oral and head and neck cancer almost always produces a series of side effects that range from the merely bothersome to some that can be severely debilitating and affect overall cancer management and quality of life. Often, there is the immediate need to begin treatment without mention or discussion of specific side effects that each patient may be facing. These could be related to the surgical management as a stand-alone treatment or surgery in combination with radiation therapy and or chemotherapy. The increasing use of chemotherapy in the management of certain forms of head and neck cancer carries its own set of possible or anticipated adverse effects.

The oral complications or side effect profile of head and neck cancer management vary widely from patient to patient and according to the treatment rendered, ranging from mild and temporary to severe and long-lasting, even lifelong in many cases. With this in mind, the routine management of the mouth and the teeth becomes an important issue in an ongoing way, with the patient's dental care provider being a critical member of the management team along with the cancer surgeon, radiation oncologist, medical oncologist, speech and swallowing therapists, and others. In cases where surgically created anatomical deficits are present, a maxillofacial prosthodontist will also be involved.

Surgical Management

When surgery alone is the treatment rendered for relatively limited or stage 1 and 2 cancers, post-treatment dental and oral management may be almost routine in nature. In cases where a surgically created deficit may result in speech alteration, the patient may require the services of a trained speech pathologist. When a swallowing deficit or difficulty is encountered, specialized tests may be needed to identify the specific reason for the dysfunction, with swallowing therapy to follow, along with a modified diet until the results of therapy will permit the patient to consume a wider range of foods.

When removal of a portion of the upper or lower jaw is a component of the surgical management, the issue of reconstruction becomes an issue. This complex area of care often relies on coordination of several providers including the cancer surgeon, the reconstructive surgeon and a maxillofacial prosthodontist. The collective goal is the restoration of function and esthetics of the jaws and the orofacial complex. This may relate to use of specialized techniques of oral appliance design, the possible use of dental implants to help stabilize and retain appliances that will be fabricated to seal off the surgically created upper jaw defects (an obturator), or removable devices to allow chewing, enhance facial esthetics and support of the face. Bone grafting techniques, including harvesting of associated bone and muscle, with its own blood supply, from other parts of the body, can be placed into the surgical defects, and connected to local arteries and veins to preserve the viability of the grafted tissue. The grafted bone will act as the missing segment of jaw and may later be restored by a maxillofacial prosthodontist to regain chewing function and facial esthetics.

Radiation Therapy

Dental input and intervention as it concerns the delivery of radiation treatment is ideally established when the decision is made to undergo this option of treatment. Most radiation oncologists integrate the dental component of care on a routine basis, referring the cancer patient for a dental evaluation prior to initiating radiation therapy. Necessary extractions are performed allowing preliminary healing in advance of radiation therapy.

Once the dental evaluation is completed and radiation treatment is underway, a rigorous oral care prevention regimen must be developed. The dentist should carefully explain to the patient the importance of this lifelong regimen as it relates to the side effects of radiation therapy and its long-term effects. The patient should be aware of the early side effects of head and neck radiation therapy that are likely to include radiation-induced dry mouth (xerostomia) and mouth and throat soreness (mucositis). The imminent reduction of saliva flow may likely produce several functional problems, as well, including difficulty in eating, swallowing, and some speech alterations.

As a result of the dry mouth, the twice-daily application of high-strength fluoride becomes mandatory in an effort to prevent the rapid onset of dryness-associated dental decay. This application can be accomplished by the use of a tray appliance or mouth guard within which fluoride gel is placed. Alternatively, some practitioners prefer to use the same form of fluoride on the toothbrush instead of toothpaste on a twice-daily basis in place of trays. Neutral sodium fluoride, 5,000 parts per million or stannous fluoride, 0.4% are recommended and should be discussed with the dentist or dental hygienist. In addition, the use of over the counter fluoride rinses are available and are often recommended to supplement high-strength fluoride gels.

When using trays, a thin layer of fluoride is placed into the tray and placed over the teeth for 10 minutes, avoiding swallowing excess fluoride following routine brushing. After removal of the trays they should be washed under cold water and stored in a cool well-ventilated place. It is recommended that the patient not eat or rinse for 30 minutes after the trays are removed. If it is not feasible to use high-strength fluoride in trays, brushing with high-strength fluoride gel can be performed twice daily.

To combat the problem of reduction or absence of saliva, two commonly prescribed drugs are available-cevimeline (Evoxac) and pilocarpine (Salagen). Stimulation of saliva with sugar-free candy or chewing gum is often helpful, as are saliva substitutes in the form of sprays and gels, which are available over the counter. Over time, some return of saliva production may be noticed, but rarely to preradiation levels.

The rationale for an aggressive and necessary dental prevention program concerns itself with avoiding the need for dental extractions in the years to come due to decay or periodontal (gum) disease. If an oral surgical procedure is necessary, there is a significant risk of developing a condition known as osteoradionecrosis (bone death due to radiation). This condition, resulting from a reduction of blood flow and fibrosis within the jaw secondary to radiation therapy is permanent. As a result of less blood flow to the jaw, any tooth extraction site may not heal properly and may become infected, thus characterizing osteoradionecrosis.

Management of this complication may include administration of hyperbaric oxygen therapy before and after a planned extraction in an effort to increase the number of new blood vessels in the area, thus promoting healing without infection and without bone becoming necrotic or dying (osteoradionecrosis). If osteonecrosis develops, a similar treatment with hyperbaric oxygen precedes removal of dead bone, followed again with a second course of hyperbaric treatment. However, this treatment may not be universally available and may not be covered by some insurance plans.

Although most dental providers are aware of cancer treatment and the effects of radiation therapy on the mouth, salivary glands, and teeth, some might not be aware of managing the complications. If this is the case, most radiation oncologists and head and neck surgeons should be able to assist in the proper referral.

Other forms of radiation-induced oral complications include altered, diminished, or loss of taste sensation and radiation-induced mucositis or mouth and throat sores. Although little can be done regarding taste alterations, there may be a return of this sense in the months following treatment. Treatment for mucositis may include salt water and baking soda rinses, topical anesthetics, compounded rinses containing combinations of a topical anesthetic, a soothing liquid such as milk of magnesia, and a flavoring agent. Several commercially available or over-the-counter nonalcoholic mouth rinses may be helpful (Oasis, Crest pro-Health, Biotene) as well. A comprehensive listing of many products is found in Chapter 16.

During the early phases of radiation therapy actual dental treatment short of tooth extractions and bony periodontal surgery can proceed normally. Performance of routine cleanings (prophylaxis procedures), fillings, bridgework, and removable dentures are permissible without any increased level of precautions. The issue of dental implant placement in the irradiated jaw following strict protocol (including hyperbaric oxygen therapy) has been studied with good long-term results after prosthetic replacement. Implants may also be placed in bone grafts as well, in association with the hyperbaric oxygen treatment to be considered in either the irradiated native jaw bone or bone that is imported to the jaw from elsewhere (usually the fibula or leg bone).

Maintenance of oral moisture is often a problem; in particular, when radiation therapy includes the salivary glands within the treatment field. The patient may need to modify his or her diet with the addition of softer or blended foods until salivary function improves. Small bites of food that are lukewarm or cool and avoidance of abrasive and highly spiced foods are often necessary. Special cookbooks are available for the oral and head and neck cancer patient that suggest a wide range of foods and recipes that are more tolerable and nutritionally sound. If eating a normal or modified diet is not yet possible, calorie and protein intake can be achieved with liquid products such as Boost, Ensure, Scandishake, and others. Lubricants such as aloe vera or lanolin on the lips may be helpful.

Some consideration may be given to the use of remineralizing solutions to help stop the process of calcium loss from the teeth in areas of very early decay. The treated patient must be aware of the fact that he or she will be susceptible to dental decay at a much higher level than before treatment as a result of mouth dryness and the loss of the natural protective substances that saliva contains; therefore, the frequency of dental visits will be greater than before treatment. As an extension of the prevention strategy, consideration must be given to performing any dental procedures as early as possible.

Chemotherapy

The emerging role of chemotherapy in the management of oral and head neck cancer has heightened the risk of treatment-induced mucositis. Although the mechanism of mucositis production differs from that due to radiation therapy, the result is essentially the same and will be considered collectively. This side effect can be heightened or amplified when radiation therapy is also a component of overall management.

Severe mucositis can be present in upward of 90% of head and neck cancer patients receiving chemoradiotherapy, thus imposing an additional burden on quality of life and resources. Management of this problem remains difficult, with several agents now in clinical trial. The traditional approaches with topical lidocaine and orally administered analgesics including opioids for pain are only marginally effective as are salt water/bicarbonate rinses. Recent preliminary studies using low energy laser therapy reduced symptoms dramatically. Additionally, studies employing the use of the growth factors, palifermin and velifermin, have shown great promise, in particular, when considered in a combined manner with laser treatment. Final recommendations await the completion of further clinical studies concerning these modalities.

Post-Treatment Care

Maintenance of teeth, jawbone integrity, and any dental appliances becomes a permanent or lifelong consideration. Prevention of infection of the supporting oral structures and gum tissues and maintaining tooth integrity and overall dental health is crucial. To help accomplish this, dental care must be extended beyond what may have been the case before cancer treatment was undertaken. Routine follow-up and maintenance with the dentist, dental hygienist, and prosthodontist is an absolute requirement that will be more frequent than anytime previously.

The patient should inform any new dental provider not familiar with his or her cancer diagnosis and treatment that he or she has had chemotherapy or radiation therapy. This may result in adjustment of care and formulation of a treatment plan that will include a more aggressive preventive strategy and increased follow-up visits.

Good follow-up care is essential in cases where dental appliances, such as obturators, are in place. This type of appliance seals off the nasal cavity and paranasal sinuses from the mouth allowing normal chewing, swallowing, and speech as well as esthetic appearance. Dental implants may be used to retain or hold the obturator or removable devices firmly in place if teeth are absent or are inadequate for proper obturator stability and function, whereas other circumstances will allow the remaining teeth to act as anchoring points. The complexity of some devices and appliances usually requires the services of a maxillofacial prosthodontist for appliance fabrication and adjustment as well as long-term maintenance.

By far the most important aspect of dental health preservation, dental restorations and appliance longevity is faithful adherence to home-care measures. These measures include careful use of dental floss before brushing and use of fluoride-containing toothpaste or dental trays as stated earlier. Use of regular toothpaste without whiteners and tartar control formulation is encouraged. If brushing after meals is not possible, rinsing with water should be done. Avoid use of excessively flavored or "spicy" flavors such as those containing cinnamon or cinnamon flavoring that may cause burning of the mouth lining.

In summary, the adherence to rigorous daily and ongoing dental and oral care and responsible dietary habits during and following cancer treatment is essential. Early communication with the entire management team from the hospital to community practices and required follow-up care and vigilance on a routine basis will help ensure a continuous level of oral health and function.

Further Reading

Chambers, M. S., Garden, A. S., Kies, M. S., & Martin, J. W. (2004). Radiation-induced xerostomia in patients with head and neck cancer: Pathogenesis, impact on quality of life, and management. *Head and Neck, 26,* 796–807.

Chiapasco, M., Biglioli, F., Autelitano, L., Romeo, E., & Brusati, R. (2006). Clinical outcome of dental implants placed in fibula-free flaps for the reconstruction of maxillo-mandibular defects following ablation for tumors or osteoradionecrosis. *Clinical Oral Implants Research*, *17*, 220–228.

Donoff, R. B. (2006). Treatment of the irradiated patient with dental implants: The case against hyperbaric oxygen treatment. *Journal of Oral and Maxillofacial Surgery*, *64*, 819–822.

Duke, R. L., Campbell, B. H., Indresano, A. T., Eaton, D. J., Marbella, A. M., Myers, K. B., . . . Layde, B. M. (2005). Dental status and quality of life in long-term head and neck cancer survivors. *Laryngoscope*, *115*, 678–683.

Granstrom, G. (2006). Placement of dental implants in irradiated bone: The case for using hyperbaric oxygen. *Journal of Oral and Maxillofacial Surgery*, *64*, 812–818.

Kielbassa, A. M., Hinkelbein, W., Hellwig, E., & Meyer-Lackel, H. (2006). Radiation-related damage to dentition. *Lancet Oncology*, *7*, 326–335.

Miller, E. H., & Quinn, A. I. (2006). Dental considerations in the management of head and neck cancer patients. *Otolaryngologic Clinics of North America*, *39*, 319–332.

Omer, O., MacCarthy, D., Nunn, J., & Cotter, E. (2005). Oral health needs of the head and neck radiotherapy patient: 2. Oral and dental care before, during and after radiotherapy. *Dental Update*, *32*, 575–576, 578–580, 582.

Peled, M., El-Naaj, I. A., Lipin, Y., & Ardekian, L. (2005). The use of free fibular flap for functional mandibular reconstruction. *Journal of Oral and Maxillofacial Surgery*, *63*, 220–224.

For Additional Information

Head and Neck Cancer: Questions and Answers.
http://www.Cancer.gov/cancertopics/factsheet/
Sites-Types/head-and-neck

E-mail: cancergovstaff@mail.nih.gov

Call: NCI Cancer Information Service at
1-800-4-Cancer (1-800-422-6237)

8

MEETING THE CHALLENGES OF TARGETED THERAPY AND SKIN CARE

Mario E. Lacouture, MD

Cancer Treatments and the Skin

Anticancer treatments such as chemotherapy and radiation owe their effectiveness to an interference with rapidly growing cells (a hallmark of cancer). This explains the frequent occurrence of side effects in normal tissues that are also composed of rapidly growing cells, such as the skin, hair, and nails. In particular, the newly introduced targeted therapies result in distinctive dermatologic side effects that may affect quality of life and in some cases result in treatment interruption or discontinuation. Interestingly, these new targeted therapies are directed at specific receptor molecules of cancer cells and may produce fewer side effects than conventional chemotherapy, where nearly all cells and tissues are affected in a relatively indiscriminate fashion; which makes the significance of dermatological side effects resulting from targeted therapies greatly heightened (Balagula et al., 2011).

Improvements in chemotherapy and radiation have allowed for more precise "targeting" of tumor cells, resulting in minimal or no side effects to bone marrow and internal organs. This has allowed for better clinical responses leading to longer survival. Treatments that are "targeted" offer the promise of a more favorable safety profile. This is partly a result of their ability to affect molecules that are pivotal in cancer cell growth. Coincidentally, one of the primary receptor molecules involved in head and neck squamous cell carcinoma (HNSCC) is known as the epidermal growth factor receptor (EGFR). This receptor is targeted by cetuximab (Erbitux), which has been approved by the U.S. Food and Drug Administration (FDA, 2007) for the treatment of HNSCC in combination with radiation (http://www.fda.gov).

The skin is composed of three major layers: the epidermis (outermost layer), which is composed of rapidly growing cells; the underlying layer (dermis), which contains nerves, blood vessels, and hair follicles and provides structural support; and the deeper fatty layer (or hypodermis), which protects against cold temperature and trauma. Thus, the close proximity and similarity of the skin to tissues affected by HNSCC make it a categorical "innocent bystander" subject to the effects of radiation therapy and targeted anticancer drugs. Efforts to reduce the impact of cancer treatments on the skin should be implemented early. Patients' knowledge of side effects and their early reporting to the oncology team will help to ensure that consistent anticancer treatment and quality of life are maintained and that the maximum benefit from therapy is gained.

Targeted Anticancer Treatments and the Skin

The EGFR is required for normal skin, hair, and nail growth and overall health (King, Gates, Stoscheck, & Nanney, 1990). Consequently, when its activity is blocked, cells are unable to function properly, resulting in skin inflammation or rash, abnormal growth, tenderness, or itching and raising the possibility of infection (Lacouture, 2006). The potentially serious dermatological side effects resulting from targeted therapies may impact the treatment of HNSCC as they may lead to modification of the use of the anticancer treatment drug as reported in 17% of patients or its permanent discontinuation in approximately 4% of patients (Bonner et al., 2006).

Drugs targeting the EGFR have also been approved in the treatment of other tumors, such as colorectal, lung, and pancreatic cancers. Considerable information has been collected on the appearance and management of dermatologic side effects in these other settings. Whereas these observations may give some insight into the development of side effects in patients with HNSCC, they must not be applied directly in this setting for two reasons. First, in HNSCC, EGFR-targeting drugs, when given with radiation therapy, are usually used for a short period of time (approximately 8 weeks) whereas in other cancers, when given alone, they are used indefinitely, creating a new set of side effects (Lacouture, Hwang, Marymont, & Patel, 2007; Roe et al., 2006). Second, the sequence in which radiation therapy is administered to head and neck cancer patients also affects the way in which the side effects appear in the skin. Thus, radiation therapy given prior to a targeted therapy will result in the sparing of EGFR-targeting drug-induced rash (Bossi et al., 2007), and radiation therapy given concurrently with drug therapy will result in the worsening of rash in the radiated areas such as the neck region.

Another class of drugs frequently used in HNSCC is the taxane group. In particular, docetaxel (Taxotere) can cause skin and nail changes in up to 80% of people. An itchy rash affecting the scalp and backs of the hands or feet can occur in up to 30% of people. Although usually mild, it can be relieved with topical corticosteroids (Elocon or Lidex creams, available with a prescription from your doctor). Nail changes are probably the most important side effect, since they affect the ability to do daily chores in up to 30% of people, and nail infections can occur in 25% of people treated with Taxotere. Once the nails have separated, it is important to keep the area dry and to prevent infections. Some studies suggest that vitamin B7 (biotin, 2.5 mg or 2,500 micrograms a day) can speed up nail growth, so it may be a good time to start taking this vitamin.

If nail infections secondary to Taxotere use have developed (you can tell by pain under the nails, sometimes with smelly fluid leaking from the nails), your doctor will probably prescribe an antibiotic after obtaining a culture. It is also a good idea to soak your fingers and toes in a solution of white vinegar in lukewarm tap water (equal amounts) for 15 minutes every evening, to help kill the bacteria and dry the nail beds. Your doctor may also recommend the use of cold gloves and socks (Elasto Gel Cold Therapy Gloves and Socks) during each Taxotere infusion. The idea is that the cold will cause blood vessels to shrink in your hands and feet, thereby decreasing the amount of Taxotere delivered to your nails, decreasing the side effects by up to four times (Scotté et al., 2005, Scotté et al., 2007).

Side Effects of Treatment on Skin

The most frequent and clinically significant side effects from the use of EGFR-targeting drugs occur in the skin. A rash affecting the face, scalp, and upper trunk will appear in as many as 87%

of patients receiving cetuximab (Erbitux) and may be associated with itching or tenderness. The majority of these cases are mild to moderate, but as many as 17% of cases may be severe and require the modification of the drug due to discomfort and possible skin infection. It is noteworthy that, although the rash may look like acne, for which it has been incorrectly labeled "acneiform"; it is not acne and does not respond to most topical acne medications.

The rash appears within the first few weeks after the first infusion of the drug and is characterized by several phases (Lacouture, 2006). In the first, occurring within the initial days, a sensation of sunburn with swelling of the nose predominates. If prophylactic treatment against rash has not already taken place, it is advisable to inform the oncologist or oncology nurse so that treatment can be initiated to prevent progression to a more severe grade. In the next phase, which occurs at the end of the first week or beginning of the 2nd week, red-yellow bumps appear on the skin, which may bleed and itch. Overall the size and number of bumps tend to peak in the 2nd to 3rd week, then slowly decrease in severity, but may still require treatment. These bumps are not indicative of infection and will not be spread to other people. At the end of the third or fourth weeks, a crust forms in the areas where the bumps are located. Finally, after the rash has resolved, redness of the face ensues, leaving some areas with dilated blood vessels.

An important correlation has been observed in which those patients who develop a very bad rash have a better response in terms of the cancer and longer survival (Perez-Soler & Saltz, 2005). This remarkable connection underscores the notion that people that develop rash should be maintained on EGFR-inhibitor treatment because they are the ones that could benefit the most. Notwithstanding this fact, those who do not develop rash should not be discouraged, as excellent responses have also been observed in the absence of the rash as well.

Other skin side effects that appear after the 2nd to 4th week include dry and itchy skin. This side effect has been reported in

15% of those patients treated, with 30% of these patients report-ing dry and itchy skin of the fingertips and heels of the feet, resulting in paper-cut fissures causing tenderness and stinging (Roe et al., 2006).

Side Effects on Hair

Hair loss, as seen with conventional chemotherapy, is not charac-teristic of EGFR-targeting drugs. However, hair loss can develop in as many as 4% of patients and tends to occur after 4 to 6 months of continuous EGFR-targeted treatment. It usually affects only the front of the scalp (as seen in older men). On the other hand, the rash that occurs on the face in the first few weeks can extend beyond the face and upper trunk and may involve the scalp, leading to itchy bumps along with hair loss. Exceptional growth of eyelashes and facial hair has been observed in 6% of treated patients (Robert et al., 2005). The texture of the hair may also change, appearing more brittle and curlier as time goes on. Overall, hair problems may appear several months after treatment and are not likely to occur in the 2-month course of HNSCC therapy.

Side Effects on Nails

After the sixth week of treatment, inflammation and redness around the fingernails and toenails occur in about 40% of patients (Roe et al., 2006). This inflammation around the nails is known as paronychia and may impair the ability to perform daily activities, such as grooming, buttoning clothes, or handling objects because of the associated tenderness. It is very important that the health care team be informed at the first sign of this effect (redness, tenderness, or fraying of the cuticles). Brittle nails may also appear, although infrequently.

Radiation Therapy and the Skin

Despite remarkable advances in radiation oncology, radiodermatitis (skin inflammation, with redness, swelling, and pain) remains a common side effect of radiation therapy. In the study that led to the FDA's approval of treatment using cetuximab combined with radiotherapy, 86% of patients receiving combined treatment suffered from radiodermatitis, of which 23% of the cases were considered severe (Bonner et al., 2006). Notably, in the absence of cetuximab, this side effect was seen in a similar number of patients treated with radiation alone. However, anecdotal reports (Budach, Böieke, & Home, 2007) and clinical experience at a large-volume referral center, the SERIES (Skin and Eye Reactions to Inhibitors of EGFR and kinaseS) Clinic (Lacouture, Basti, Patel, & Benson, 2006),suggests that combining Erbitux and radiation therapy may lead to more severe radiodermatitis (Tejwani et al., 2009). More studies are needed to confirm this observation, and this should be set in the context that this combination led to significantly greater anticancer activity than either therapy alone.

Prevention and Treatment of Dermatologic Side Effects

There are two key elements that help to minimize the impact of dermatological side effects on quality of life: (a) early recognition of the side effects so that prompt treatments can be instituted, and (b) the use of treatments tailored to the location and type of side effect. A proactive approach dictates that therapy begin before the onset of anticancer treatment limiting the chances of development of skin effects and their severity. This is an approach that has already shown promise in the treatment of rash to EGFR-inhibitor drugs. Knowledge of the sequence of side effect development is critical to anticipating these dermatologic side effects: rash (weeks 1 to 3), nail inflammation (weeks 2 to 6), dry skin (weeks 6 to 8), and hair problems (weeks 12 to 24) (Lynch et al., 2007).

Several measures can be initiated prior to or when therapy is started:

- Use of a broad-spectrum sunscreen (containing zinc oxide or titanium dioxide) with an SPF (sun protection factor) of at least 15
- Use of mild soaps for showering or bathing (Dove, Cetaphil, Basis)
- Use of detergents that are free of fragrances or perfumes (All Free Clear, Tide Free)
- Use of lukewarm instead of hot water in the shower or bath
- Use of moisturizers containing ammonium lactate (Am-Lactin) or 10% urea daily, especially on very dry areas of the hands and feet (*NOT* in areas of radiation or the face).
- Use of zinc oxide containing creams (Desitin Maximum Strength) applied up to four times a day or liquid bandages (New-Skin, Liquid Band-Aids), for cracks in the fingertips or heels,
- Avoidance of sun exposure, and wearing a broad-brimmed hat
- Use of prophylactic therapy with prescription creams or oral tetracycline antibiotics when receiving cetuximab (Erbitux).
- Avoidance of tight-fitting shoes or trauma around the toenails
- Use of creams or ointments more than 4 hours before or 4 hours after radiation.
- Use of Elocon cream daily. This cream has been shown to decrease the itch and irritation associated with radiation
- If there are any signs of infection (yellow crusting, pain, fluid discharge), notify your doctor so that appropriate antibiotics may be given.
- Have contact information of the oncologist or oncology nurse available in the event they are needed.

Ask your doctor about preventing rash to cetuximab (Erbitux) with the use of topical steroids (alclometasone cream) and oral antibiotics (doxycycline or minocycline 100 mg twice daily) during the first 6 weeks.

If the rash develops, the doctor may prescribe a corticosteroid or antibiotic cream, which is to be applied thinly and evenly on the face, chest and upper back, or other affected areas. If the scalp is affected, the dermatologist may suggest foams or shampoos containing corticosteroids. Corticosteroids work by blocking inflammation, a key element in rash formation, itching, and tenderness. In some cases topical steroids (hydrocortisone or alclometasone) and oral antibiotics (doxycycline or minocycline) may be prescribed to reduce the severity of the rash. This medication should be taken on a daily basis (Lacouture et al., 2010; Scope et al., 2007).

Treatment of rash has been shown to lead to more complete improvement when it is mild in severity. Consequently, informing the doctor at this mild stage is important to achieving good results. The same principle is applied for radiodermatitis. Studies have shown that prophylactic treatment with topical steroids minimizes the severity and discomfort associated with this reaction (Bostrom, Lindman, Swartling, Berne, & Bergh, 2001). Keep in mind, however, that although it is safe to use topical steroid creams for radiodermatitis, these should be wiped off before radiation therapy is administered to minimize augmentation of energy in those areas.

As discussed previously, nail inflammation is not common in patients with HNSCC. If redness, pain, or swelling occurs despite adequate moisturization as indicated earlier, it is important to avoid infection. Soaking the tips of fingers or toes in a solution of white vinegar diluted 1:1 with water provides antiseptic relief. If drainage from areas around the nail occurs, oral antibiotic therapy may be needed (Fox, 2007). For severely dry skin, the doctor may prescribe exfoliants to remove flaking and scaling skin (e.g. ammonium lactate 12% creams (La-Hydrin or Am-Lactin, or salicylic acid (Salex 6% cream). Always try creams on a small (quarter-size) area of skin so that if irritation occurs, it is not as severe. For management of itching, use a cream that is also anti-itch (Sarna Ultra cream or Pramoxine 1% (Itch-X, ProctoFoam spray). For more severe itching, lidocaine 4% or pramoxine 1% is a good option but should be limited to smaller areas because it contains the anesthetic lidocaine. Patients with itching report immediate relief by keeping these creams in the refrigerator because they provide an immediate cooling effect when applied.

Sometimes, oral medicines against itching may be needed, such as antihistamines (for example cetirizine (Zyrtec), fexofenadine (Allegra), diphenhydramine (Benadryl), and gabapentin (Neurontin) or pregabalin (Lyrica), which may cause drowsiness, so taking them at night will provide a better night's sleep (Porzio et al., 2006).

In the great majority of cases, dermatological side effects from radiation therapy and novel targeted drugs will not lead to long-term sequelae, and anticancer treatments will not need to be modified. This can be achieved by following several principles: by employing preventive measures and initiating treatments to offset side effects as early as possible, and by patients playing an active role in treatment to get the most benefit from therapy and maintaining an optimal sense of well-being.

References

Balagula, Y., Garbe, C., Myskowski, P. L., Hauschild, A., Rapoport, B. L., Boers-Doets, C. B., & Lacouture M. E. (2011). Clinical presentation and management of dermatological toxicities of epidermal growth factor receptor inhibitors. *International Journal of Dermatology, 50*(2), 129–146. doi: 10.1111/j.1365-4632.2010.04791.x. PubMed PMID: 21244375.

Bonner, J. A., Harari, P. M., Giralt, J., Azarnia, N., Shin, D. M., Cohen, R. B., . . . Ang, K. K. (2006). Radiotherapy plus cetuximab for squamous-cell carcinoma of the head and neck. *New England Journal of Medicine, 354,* 567–578.

Bossi, P., Liberatoscioli, C., Bergamini, C., Locati, L., Fava, S., Rinaldi, G., . . . Licitra L. (2007). Previously irradiated areas spared from skin toxicity induced by cetuximab in six patients: Implications for the administration of EGFR inhibitors in previously irradiated patients. *Annals of Oncology, 18,* 601–602.

Bostrom, A., Lindman, H., Swartling, C., Berne, B., & Bergh, J. (2001). Potent corticosteroid cream (mometasone furoate) significantly reduces acute radiation dermatitis: Results from a double-blind, randomized study. *Radiotherapy and Oncology, 59*, 257–265.

Budach, W., Bölke, E., & Homey, B. (2007). Severe cutaneous reaction during radiation therapy with concurrent cetuximab. *New England Journal of Medicine, 357*(5), 514–515.

Federal Food and Drug Association. (2007). Erbitux approval summary. Retrieved July 15, 2007, from http://www.fda.gov

Fox, L. P. (2007). Nail toxicity associated with epidermal growth factor receptor inhibitor therapy. *Journal of the American Academy of Dermatology, 56*(3), 460–465.

King, L. E., Jr., Gates, R. E., Stoscheck, C. M., & Nanney, L. B. (1990). The EGF/TGF alpha receptor in skin. *Journal of Investigative Dermatology, 94*(Suppl. 6), 164S–170S.

Lacouture, M. E. (2006). Mechanisms of cutaneous toxicities to EGFR inhibitors. *Nature Reviews Cancer, 6*, 803–812.

Lacouture, M. E., Basti, S., Patel, J., & Benson, A., 3rd. (2006). The SERIES clinic: An interdisciplinary approach to the management of toxicities of EGFR inhibitors. *Journal of Supportive Oncology, 4*, 236–238.

Lacouture, M. E., Hwang, C., Marymont, M. H., & Patel, J. (2007). Temporal dependence of the effect of radiation on erlotinib-induced skin rash. *Journal of Clinical Oncology, 25*, 2140.

Lacouture M. E., Mitchell, E. P., Piperdi, B., Pillai, M. V., Shearer, H., Iannotti, N., . . . Yassine, M. (2010). Skin toxicity evaluation protocol with panitumumab (STEPP), a phase II, open-label, randomized trial evaluating the impact of a pre-Emptive Skin Treatment regimen on skin toxicities and quality of life in patients with metastatic colorectal cancer. *Journal of Clinical Oncology, 28*(8), 1351–1357. Epub 2010 Feb 8. PubMed PMID: 20142600. 1111/j.1365-4632.2010.04791.x. PubMed PMID: 21244375.

Lynch, T. J., Kim, E. S., Eaby, B., Garey, J., West, D. P., & Lacouture M. E. (2007). Epidermal growth factor receptor inhibitor-associated cutaneous toxicities: An evolving paradigm in clinical management. *Oncologist, 12*(5), 610–621.

Perez-Soler, R., & Saltz, L. (2005). Cutaneous adverse effects with HER1/EGFR-targeted agents: Is there a silver lining? *Journal of Clinical Oncology, 23*, 5235–5246.

Porzio, G., Aielli, F., Verna, L., Porto, C., Tudini, M., Cannita, K., . . . (2006). Efficacy of pregabalin in the management of cetuximab-related itch. *Journal of Pain and Symptom Management, 32*, 397–398.

Robert, C., Soria, J. C., Spatz, A., Le Cesne, A., Malka, D., Pautier, P., . . . Le Chavelier, T. (2005). Cutaneous side-effects of kinase inhibitors and blocking antibodies. *Lancet Oncology, 6*, 491–500.

Roe, E., Garcia Muret, M. P., Marcuello, E., Capdevila, J., Pallares, C., & Alomar, A. (2006). Description and management of cutaneous side effects during cetuximab or erlotinib treatments: A prospective study of 30 patients. *Journal of the American Academy of Dermatology*, *55*, 429–437.

Scope, A., Agero, A. L., Dusza, S. W., Myskowski, P. L., Lieb, J. A., Saltz, L., . . . (2007). Randomized double-blind trial of prophylactic oral minocycline and topical tazarotene for cetuximab-associated acne-like eruption. *Journal of Clinical Oncology*, *25*(34), 5390–5396.

Scotté, F., Banu, E., Medioni, J., Levy, E., Ebenezer, C., Marsan, S., . . . Oudard S. (2008). Matched case-control phase 2 study to evaluate the use of a frozen sock to prevent docetaxel-induced onycholysis and cutaneous toxicity of the foot. *Cancer*, *112*(7), 1625–1631. PubMed PMID: 18286527.

Scotté, F., Tourani, J. M., Banu, E., Peyromaure, M., Levy, E., Marsan, S., . . . Oudard, S. (2005). Multicenter study of a frozen glove to prevent docetaxel-induced onycholysis and cutaneous toxicity of the hand. *Journal of Clinical Oncology*, *23*(19), 4424-4429. PubMed PMID:15994152.

Tejwani, A., Wu, S., Jia, Y., Agulnik, M., Millender, L., & Lacouture, M. E. (2009). Increased risk of high-grade dermatologic toxicities with radiation plus epidermal growth factor receptor inhibitor therapy. *Cancer*, *115*(6), 1286–1299. PubMed PMID: 19170238.

9

MEETING THE CHALLENGES OF PAIN IN THE HEAD AND NECK CANCER PATIENT POPULATION: CAUSES AND EFFECTS

Barbara A. Murphy, MD

Introduction to Pain

Basic Anatomy

Pain is defined as a perception of an unpleasant sensation. In order to maximize pain control it is important to understand the underlying biology. There are nerve cells located throughout the body that are designed specifically to detect signals indicating damage or potential damage to tissues. These nerve cells have endings that detect different types of tissue damage. For example, there are special nerve endings that are able to detect heat, others are able to detect pressure, and still others are able to detect tissue inflammation due to a wound or infection. These nerves are part of what is called the *peripheral* nervous system. If a nerve ending is activated, it sends an impulse along the nerve to the spinal cord. The spinal cord acts as a highway by which impulses from the peripheral nervous system are processed and the pain signal is directed toward the brain. Once the signal reaches the brain, we perceive and react to the pain. The nerves in the spinal cord and the brain are considered part of the *central* nervous system.

Communicating with the Health Care Team

Good pain control requires **good communication** between patients and health care providers. Pain is a complicated symptom. In order to address pain adequately, providers need sufficient information to guide their treatment decisions. The following section provides a basic knowledge about pain to aid communication with the health care team (Wells et al., 2003). It is critical to know who will be providing care for pain and pain related problems. Questions to ask your health care providers include:

- Who will be responsible for writing prescriptions for pain medications?
- Who will be responsible for making changes to the pain treatment regimen?
- What is the best way to contact that individual?

Types of Pain

There are two general types of pain: nociceptive and neuropathic. Nociceptive pain occurs when there is normal activation
of a pain receptor and the signal is transmitted via the nerves to
the brain. This type of pain may be described as aching, throb-
bing, deep, or squeezing. Neuropathic pain is caused by damage
to nerves or nerve endings. The damaged nerve fires pain signals
to the brain in an abnormal manner. Neuropathic pain is usually
described as sharp, stabbing, or burning pain. It is important to
distinguish these two types of pain because they have very different causes and because they are often treated differently.

Time Course of Pain

Pain may be brief and of short duration. We call this type of pain
"acute." It often can be attributed to an easily identified cause.
For example, ankle pain after a sprain is "acute pain." Pain may
also be recurrent or persistent for prolonged periods of time.
For example, many patients with arthritis of the knees experience constant joint pain. This is called "chronic" pain. Acute and
chronic pain can occur at the same time. For example, a patient
with chronic knee pain due to arthritis may experience acute
worsening of pain in cold weather. It is very important to relay
information about the time course to the health care providers.
It may help them determine the type of pain, its cause, and how
to treat it. Important questions include:

■ When did the pain first start?
■ How long has it lasted?
■ Does it get better or worse at different times?

Functional Pain

There are times when patients will experience pain only when
they perform specific tasks. For example, patients with back
pain may say that their pain is controlled when they lie down,
but when they stand or walk the pain is worse. This is called

functional pain. Functional pain can be very difficult to treat because pain medications may only be needed sporadically or the pain may not respond well to pain medications. Functional pain is common in head and neck cancer patients. For example, the pain due to mucositis (inflammation of the lining of the mouth and throat) worsens with swallowing. Specific information that patients should give their provider includes:

- What type of activity makes the pain worse?
- What makes the pain feel better?

Severity of Pain

When discussing pain, health care providers will ask about the severity of pain. Keeping track of this information using a daily diary may help patients and health care providers direct changes in pain medications. Most often pain is graded on a scale of 0 to 10. Zero means no pain and 10 means excruciating pain. Specific questions that are asked about pain intensity include the following:

- The current pain level
- The average pain level
- The worst pain level on a daily basis
- The pain level after taking pain medications.

Pain Frequency

Pain may occur now and again (intermittent) or it may be present all the time (constant). If pain is intermittent, patients are instructed to take their pain medications "as needed." That means that if pain begins to develop, patients are instructed to take their medications. If pain is constant, then patients need to take pain medication "around the clock." Around the clock means that you take medications on a routine basis. The purpose of taking pain medication "around the clock" is to keep the blood level of the pain medication at a point that is effective for controlling pain. Patients often discontinue their "around the clock" medication when their pain is controlled. This is a mistake: the blood level of the pain medication will drop and the pain will return. It is best to think of pain medication for constant pain in the same way you think of high blood pressure medications: you find the dose that controls the problem and you continue to take the medication until your doctor tells you otherwise.

Breakthrough Pain

Patients who are on "around the clock" pain medication may experience what is referred to as *"breakthrough pain."* Breakthrough pain is a sudden flare-up of pain. Patients with breakthrough pain will need a "rescue dose" of medication. "Breakthrough" or "rescue" medications are fast acting (immediate release) medications. They should take effect with 1 to 2 hours. If the medication does not work within this time period, then another dose is needed. Keeping track of the number of rescue doses is important. If patients take more than 4 rescue doses per day, the health care providers will increase the around-the-clock dosing. Health care providers will ask the following questions about breakthrough pain:

■ Are there episodes of breakthrough pain?
■ How severe is the breakthrough pain?
■ How often does the breakthrough pain occur?
■ How many rescue doses are required each day?

Pain Emergency

There are times when pain is severe and uncontrollable. When this happens, patients should contact their health care team. Often, patients will be directed to their emergency room or will be admitted to the hospital to get the pain under control. This is particularly important if pain is causing other problems such as difficulty swallowing and dehydration.

Psychology of Pain

Pain is not a simple biological process. For cancer patients and their families, pain is often associated with the cancer itself;

thus, it is an emotionally laden symptom. Often, family members will report high levels of distress when they witness pain in a loved one. Allowing family members to express their thoughts and feelings about the pain experience is important for both the patient and the family.

The current pain experience may be dramatically affected by past experiences with pain, particularly if the experience was poor. It is important for patients to communicate past pain events with the health care team so that they can work to prevent a bad past experience from affecting the current situation.

Pain may be associated with mood disorders such as depression and anxiety (Spiegel & Koopman, 1994). It should be noted that patients with mood disorders often report more pain and greater intensity of pain. It is therefore very important to treat mood disorders aggressively with medication and counseling. This is particularly important for head and neck cancer patients because they often have associated high rates of both depression and anxiety.

Pain causes both physical and emotional stress. In addition, stress may worsen the pain experience. Some patients are able to deal with stress well. They have strategies to deal with stress such as music, art, pets, or a hobby. Some patients have outside support systems that help them cope with stress. Friends, family, support groups, and religious organizations all can provide a helping hand. There are also a wealth of organizations and services dedicated to helping cancer patients cope with the difficult task of dealing with cancer. For patients who have difficulty dealing with the stress of cancer or patients who feel that stress is making pain management difficult, reaching out for help can make a huge difference.

Barriers to Good Pain Control

There are a number of barriers to good pain control. The first, poor communication has already been addressed. Perhaps the most problematic barrier to good pain control is the concern of patients, family and society at large about the use of controlled substances such as opioids (Miaskowski et al., 2001). It should be noted that unless a patient has a history of alcohol or substance abuse, it is uncommon for patients to become addicted to pain medications during the course of their cancer treatment. On the other hand, patients with a history or substance abuse are at risk for relapse if the use of opioids or other controlled substances are not administered and monitored carefully. Patients with a substance abuse history should discuss these issues openly with their health care provider to ensure that a plan is outlined to minimize the risk of relapse. Due to the inherent risk to the patient and others, opioids and other controlled substances are not prescribed for patients who are actively abusing either legal or illegal drugs.

Pain medications are expensive. Even for patients with excellent insurance, the co-payments for pain medications can be high. For patients who lack insurance or prescription drug coverage, pain medications are often beyond their capacity to afford. There are pharmaceutical companies, hospitals, and community organizations that provide assistance to patients with financial barriers to pain control. Patients should seek guidance from their health care team should finances be an issue.

Medical Issues and Pain Control

Patients should discuss their medical history with their physician prior to starting on a pain regimen. Some medical problems may impact on the patient's ability to tolerate or metabolize medications. The following is a select list of medical issues that may alter the use of pain medications:

■ Patients with kidney problems will excrete opioid breakdown products more slowly.
■ Older patients tend to excrete opioid breakdown products more slowly

■ Patients with advanced liver disease may metabolize opioids more slowly

■ Patients with a history of GI bleeding may need to avoid NSAIDs

■ Patients with diabetes should be carefully monitored if placed on steroids.

Diagnostic Testing

If the cause of pain is obvious, a treatment plan may be developed without obtaining further studies. However, when the cause of pain is unclear, a workup may be needed. In head and neck cancer patients this may include the following:

■ An endoscopic evaluation to look at the lining of the throat and mouth to identify any abnormalities

■ Imaging studies to look for evidence of tumor or treatment related issue injury

■ Neurophysiologic testing (e.g., electromyography) to evaluate the function of nerves and muscles to determine the source of pain or weakness.

Causes of Pain in Head and Neck Cancer

There are several important reasons to know the cause of a patient's pain (Vecht Hoff et al., 1991). First, pain may be caused by a reversible or treatable process. For example, head and neck cancer patients often develop fungal infections in their mouth and throat. This can easily be treated with antifungal medications. Second, different types of pain may need different types of treatment. For example, nerve pain tends to be less responsive to opioids; thus, other types of pain types medication may be required. Finally, pain may indicate a problem that requires immediate care.

Cancer as a Cause of Pain

Cancer itself may at times cause considerable pain. Pain may be the first sign of cancer and may be the complaint that brings patients to their health care providers for evaluation (Chaplin & Morton, 1999). Most often cancer related pain is due to infiltration of normal tissues by cancer cells. Head and neck cancers may also cause pain in other ways. The eustachian tube connects the middle ear with the throat. When it is blocked by cancer, fluid builds up in the middle ear causing pain and pressure. The head and neck region has an extensive supply of nerves. Cancers may invade directly into nerves or travel along nerves causing neuropathic or nerve pain. Cancers may become infected causing swelling and inflammation of the surrounding tissues. Finally, they may destroy or weaken bones resulting in painful fractures.

Treatment as a Cause of Pain

Surgery—Acute Pain

Patients who undergo surgical procedures are expected to have postoperative pain. The severity of the pain depends largely on the extent of the surgical procedure. For minor procedures, postoperative pain is usually managed by the surgeon using oral medications. For larger procedures, particularly those requiring hospitalization, the anesthesiologist or critical care specialist will work with the surgeons to maximize pain control. Spinal analgesia or intravenous pain medications may be required to optimize pain control. Generally, postoperative pain will resolve over a few days to weeks. For some patients, postoperative pain may last longer, requiring longer use of pain medications. For example, patients with a skin graft or flap reconstruction may experience more prolonged pain.

Surgery—Chronic Pain

During surgery nerves and tissues are cut; this may lead to pain that can be permanent. In addition, surgery results in the development of scar tissue. Scar tissue is hard and may contract. This may result in abnormal posture and decreased range of motion of the jaw, neck, and shoulders. Long term, this may lead to chronic pain problems. It is important for patients to tell their physician about muscular or bone pain, or problems that develop with moving the neck, shoulders or jaw (Chau et al., 1999). Referral to a physical therapist may help decrease the tightness of the tissues allowing improved range of motion, better posture, and decreased pain.

Radiation—Acute

Radiation therapy may be used alone, or in combination with chemotherapy. The two most common causes of pain due to radiation are mucositis and dermatitis. *Mucositis* is an inflammation of the lining of the mouth and throat. *Dermatitis* is an inflammation of the skin (Murphy, 2007). The severity of both of these symptoms depends on the dose of radiation, the amount of tissue being radiated, and whether chemotherapy is being given simultaneously. Simultaneous chemotherapy and radiation dramatically increases the severity of both mucositis and dermatitis.

Symptoms from mucositis usually begin the second or third week of radiation therapy. Initially patients will note mild irritation and soreness of the mouth and throat. By week 4 to 5, ulcers begin to develop causing a substantial increase in pain (Wong et al., 2006). In some patients, pain may continue to increase for two to three weeks post radiation. When mucositis begins to heal, pain usually begins to subside. Mucositis may dramatically impact on important functions such as swallowing, talking, and sleeping.

As the pain due to mucositis evolves rapidly, patients require very frequent monitoring. Initially, topical lidocaine containing solutions (a numbing medication), acetaminophen (Tylenol), anti-inflammatories (such as Motrin or Aleve), or low doses of opioids are commonly used for patients with mild pain from mucositis. As pain worsens, patients usually need to progress to stronger doses of opioids. Unfortunately, at the same time, patients' ability to swallow decreases substantially. One method for administering pain medication to patients who are unable to swallow is the use of patches containing forms of pain relievers that are absorbable through the skin. Short-acting liquid narcotics, which can be swallowed more easily or given by a feeding tube, can be used for breakthrough pain. Pain due to radiation mucositis takes weeks to months to resolve.

Radiation also causes a burn of the skin. This is usually called radiation dermatitis (inflammation of the skin due to radiation therapy). It usually begins as redness and dry cracking or peeling skin. Some patients develop more severe skin reactions with oozing, ulcerative appearing skin changes. Radiation dermatitis usually resolves within 2 to 3 weeks of completing radiation therapy. To date, no topical agents have been shown to prevent radiation dermatitis or mucous membrane inflammation (radiation mucositis) (see Chapter 16).

Radiation—Chronic

Similar to surgery, radiation can cause the development of scar tissue within the jaw, neck, and shoulders. Patients may develop abnormal posture and decreased range of motion of joints in the jaw, neck, and shoulders. Referral to a physical therapist after completion of radiation therapy is important so that patients may be instructed in exercises and stretches that may prevent these problems from developing.

After radiation mucositis has healed, patients may have persistent burning pain in their mouth and throat. This is referred to as mucosal sensitivity. Mucosal sensitivity may be made worse by spicy or acidic food, or dry air. This problem may be difficult to treat. Standard pain medications such as acetaminophen, anti-inflammatories, and opioids often fail to work in this circumstance. Topical lidocaine, ketoprofen paste, and medications that are used for nerve pain may be effective in some patients.

Chemotherapy

Specific chemotherapy agents may result in side effects that cause pain. For example, 5-fluorouracil and methotrexate, commonly used agents in head and neck cancer, routinely cause painful mucositis. In general, the mucositis is much milder than that seen with radiation therapy. Some chemotherapy drugs, such as cisplatin, may cause nerve damage. This may manifest itself as tingling, numbness, or pain. At times the nerve damage may progress and cause weakness. Vinblastine, an older chemotherapy agent that is uncommonly used today, may cause severe jaw pain during and immediately after administration.

Treatment of Pain

Basics

One of the important basics of pain control is to understand the goal of treatment. For patients with mild pain, medications may eliminate the pain totally. However, for many patients whose pain is more severe, it may not be possible to eliminate all pain. In this situation, the goal of pain medications is to "control" pain. Adequate pain control is defined by each individual patient. Pain medications often have side effects. This is particularly true for higher dose of opioids. Each patient will need to determine the best balance between their level of pain and the side effects of pain medication. Some patients would rather have the lowest possible level of pain and are willing to deal with the side effects of the pain medications. Other patients have difficulty dealing with side effects and would rather tolerate a certain level of pain. That being said, pain should be controlled as best possible because pain places severe stress on the body and decreases the functioning of the immune system. Patients should discuss these issues with their health care providers so that they can work together to find the right regimen for them.

In general, health care providers will use the mildest agent or lowest doses of medications that are effective for controlling symptoms. The World Health Organization has developed a "ladder" to help guide use of pain medications (Ventafridda et al., 1987). According to the ladder, pain is categorized as mild, moderate, or severe. Patients with mild pain are usually treated with acetaminophen or anti-inflammatory agents. If these drugs do not work or when pain is moderate, low doses of opioids are used. If low doses of opioids don't work or pain is severe, high-dose opioids are used.

This "stepped" approach to pain medication use is most effective for "nociceptive pain." Nerve pain is commonly resistant to opioids. For patients with nerve pain, alternative medications that affect ability of nerves to generate or transmit a pain signal are more effective.

In addition to medications, there are nonmedical therapies for pain. Nonmedical therapies are very diverse spanning from simple measures such as heat or cold for joint or muscles aches to relaxation techniques such as music or meditation. Use of these techniques is strongly encouraged.

Types of Pain Medications

Nonsteroidal Anti-inflammatory Agents

Aspirin and aspirin-like medications are commonly used to treat mild pain especially when pain is due to inflammation. They are very helpful for patients who have tumors involving the bones. Overall, these are safe agents when taken as directed. Side effects of these drugs include: stomach upset, stomach ulcers, damage to the kidneys and increased bleeding. For example:

Ibuprofen (Motrin) 200 to 600 mg four times a day, or 800 mg three times a day

Naproxen (Aleve) 250 to 750 mg twice a day

Diclofenac (Voltaren) 25 to 75 mg three times a day

Steroids

Steroids are potent anti-inflammatory drugs. Long-term use may cause potentially severe side effects. Therefore, they are generally used for brief periods of time to control pain due to severe inflammation and swelling. Higher dose steroids should be tapered down, rather than stopped abruptly. For example:

Prednisone or Decadron at variable doses

Acetaminophen—Tylenol

Tylenol is frequently used for mild pain. Although generally safe when taken as directed, excessive amounts of Tylenol can cause liver damage or failure. Do not take Tylenol or Tylenol-containing medications more frequently than prescribed by your doctor.

Opioids

Opioids are a type of drug that binds to the surface of receptor cells resulting in decreased pain sensation. Opioids are very effective for many patients with moderate to severe pain.

- Opioids may be given by mouth, across the skin using medication patches, under the skin, or intravenously. The method used for administering the pain medications depends on the medical issues facing individual patients. If patients are able to take medications by mouth, this route is preferred. If a patient is having difficulty swallowing, pain patches applied to the skin are a better choice. For patients with severe pain, intravenous (IV) medications may be the most effective.
- There are a number of different types of opioids available. Morphine is considered the opioid of choice by the World Health Organization because it is available in various formulations (oral short acting, oral long acting and IV), it is less expensive than many of the other opioids, and it is widely available. Other types of opioids may be chosen instead of morphine based on individual patient related issues or the preferences of the treating physician. Patients may need to switch from one opioid to another in order to find the opioid that is most effective with the least side effects. For example:

Morphine

Hydromorphone

Oxycodone

Hydrocodone

Methadone

■ Health care providers will start patients on a low dose of opioids to see if they are effective and to make sure that there are no side effects. Often, the dose of the medication will need to be increased. This is call dose "titration." If the cause of pain is treated, the dose of the opioid may be decreased or "titrated down." Patients must report the effectiveness of opioids so that the health care providers can titrate the regimen up or down as needed.

■ There are short- and long-acting opioids. Short-acting opioids have a quick time to effect (as short as 30 to 60 minutes); however, they do not last very long. Thus, they are ideal for "breakthrough medication." In addition, the dose of short-acting medications can be titrated or adjusted up very quickly if needed so they are often used in patients with new onset pain.

■ Long-acting opioids last longer so they need to be taken less frequently. However, it takes days for long-acting opioids to maximize their effect so upward titration takes longer. Because of this, short-acting opioids are often used in the initial treatment of pain in order to determine the amount needed to control pain. Once the effective dose of drug is determined, patients can switch to a long-acting form. Long-acting opioids are ideal for "around the clock" administration because they do not need to be taken too frequently. They should never be used for "breakthrough" pain.

■ In general, patients will be on a long-acting opioid for their "around the clock" pain medication and a short-acting opioid for the "breakthrough" pain.

Opioid Side Effects

Opioids frequently cause side effects. Side effects can usually be controlled. It is important that patients report side effects to their health care providers immediately so that steps can be taken to alter the treatment regimen appropriately. Patients should continue taking their opioids unless told to stop.

- *Sedation/Confusion:* Sleepiness is a common side effect of opioids. It usually gets better over time as the body "gets used" to having the medication in the system. Similarly, patients may feel a change in their thinking. They may notice a "foggy" sensation, mild confusion, a loss of mental focus, or a decrease in memory. After 3 to 10 days, these side effects usually subside as the body gets used to the medication. If a patient becomes very confused or very sleepy, **contact the health care team** immediately. Patients should be careful about driving or carrying out activities that require sharp concentration when they start opioids for pain.
- *Nausea/Vomiting:* Opioids may cause a decrease in appetite, nausea, or vomiting. If a patient develops these symptoms, contact the health care team: they can provide medications to counter the nausea and vomiting. Over time, the nausea and vomiting tends to subside.
- *Constipation:* Most patients who take opioids will develop constipation. This side effect will continue as long as the patient is on the medication. Patients should drink plenty of liquids, maintain a high-fiber diet, and remain active. If this is not sufficient to control constipation, over-the-counter and prescription laxatives are usually effective.
- *Itching:* Itching is a less common but bothersome side effect of opioids. Antihistamines such as Benadryl may decrease the symptoms.
- *Muscular Jerking (myoclonic jerks):* Patients or family members may notice a jerking of the muscles due to opioids. This is not harmful and may be treated with a number of prescription medications.

Safe and Responsible Opioid Use

Opioids are excellent medications for controlling pain. That being said, they have the potential to be misused, a common problem in our contemporary society. Misuse of opioids is usually related to prior addiction. Addiction is defined as the use of drugs in an uncontrolled, compulsive manner even in the face of harm to self. Increasingly strict rules are being imposed on health care providers, patients, and pharmaceutical companies in an effort to control this problem. It is therefore very important for patients to know their role in the safe use of opioids.

Addiction should be distinguished from physical dependence and tolerance. Patients who require long-term opioid therapy may develop physical dependence. That means that the body is accustomed to the drug. Tolerance is a decrease in the effectiveness of the drug over time. Physical dependence is common in patients who are on opioids for a long period of time. If patients discontinue their opioids suddenly, they may go into withdrawal. It is important to wean off opioids slowly to allow the body to accommodate to the decreasing doses of opioids.

The following are important pieces of information for patients to know so that they may use opioids in a safe and responsible manner.

Laws that health care providers must follow:

- Health care providers must see patients on a routine basis in order to prescribe opioids
- Opioids are generally written for a one-month supply.
- A new prescription must be written each time. Refills are not permitted.
- Opioids may not be prescribed to patients who are using illegal substances or abusing their medications.
- Some insurance providers are now requiring the following: a Control Substance Agreement signed by the patient and provider, routine urine drug screens, pill counts, and, when available, state database searches to ensure that patients are not obtaining medications from multiple health care providers. If your health care provider asks you for any of these, they are doing so in an effort to be compliant with current practice guidelines and should not be interpreted as an insult or offense.
- Pharmacies must have a "hard copy" or paper prescription for many opioid medications in order to fill them. It is important that patients plan ahead to ask for refills at their doctor's visit because these medications cannot be "called in" via telephone or fax.

Patients have the following responsibilities:

- Work with a single health care provider for pain control.
- Do not take more pain medication than has been prescribed. It is considered misuse to take opioids more frequently than prescribed. The health care provider needs to be notified if pain is uncontrolled and an increase is needed.
- Keep pain medications in a safe place.
- Keep track of the number of pills that are left in a prescription and when the prescription will run out.
- Set up a follow-up appointment in a timely manner to obtain a new prescription.
- Fill opioid prescriptions at the same pharmacy every time.
- Patients should not share their opioids with others. This is called diversion and is considered illegal.
- Patient should not use illegal drugs. If a provider does a urine drug screen and finds illegal drugs, they may be unable to prescribe further opioid pain medications.

Summary

Head and neck cancer and its treatment are associated with pain. Good pain control requires open communication between patients and health care providers about pain-related issues. Issues vary from making sure that the medication regimen is effective to addressing problems with insurance coverage. As a patient or caregiver, it is important to educate yourself about these issues so that you can be effective in communicating with your health care team. In addition, it must be recognized that pain control requires ongoing adjustments in medications. This requires patience and perseverance on the part of all those involved. That being said, good pain control can result in vast improvements in function and quality of life. Thus, the effort and time spent on managing pain is worthwhile for the patient, family, and health care providers.

References

Chaplin, J. M., & Morton, R. P. (1999). A prospective, longitudinal study of pain in head and neck cancer patients. *Head and Neck, 21,* 531–537.

Chau, K. S., Lee, M. C., & Patt, R. B. (1999). Pain and loss of function in head and neck cancer survivors. *Journal of Pain and Symptom Manage, 18*(3), 193–202.

Miaskowski, C., West, C., Paul, S. M., Tripolly, D., & Schumaker, K. (2001). Lack of adherence with the analgesic regimen: A signficanat barrier to effective cancer pain managment. *Journal of Clinical Oncology, 19,* 4275–4279.

Murphy, B. A. (2007). Clinical and economic consequences of mucositis induced by chemotherapy and/or radiation therapy. *Journal of Supportive Oncology, 5*(9, Suppl. 4), 13–21.

Spiegel, D., & Koopman, C. (1994). Pain and depression in patients with cancer. *Cancer, 74*(9), 2570–2578.

Vecht, C. J., Hoff, A. M., Kansen, P. J., de Boer, M. F., & Bosch, D. A. (1991). Types and causes of pain in cancer of the head and neck. *Cancer, 70,* 178–184.

Ventafridda, V., Carenceni, A., DeConno, F., & Naldi, F. (1987). A validation study of the WHO method for cancer pain relief. *Cancer, 59,* 850–856.

Wells, N., Murphy, B. A., Wujcik, D., & Johnson, R. (2003). Improving cancer pain managment through patient and family education. *Journal of Pain and Symptom Management, 25,* 344–356.

Wong, P. C., Dodd, M. J., Miaskowski, C., Paul, S. M., Bank, K. A., Shiba, G. H., & Facione, N. (2006). Mucositis pain induced by radiation therapy: Prevalence,severity, and use of self-care behaviors. *Journal of Pain and Symptom Management, 32*(1), 27–37.

10

MEETING THE CHALLENGES OF QUALITY OF LIFE

Dorothy Gold, MSW, LCSW-C, OSW-C

A diagnosis of cancer can be overwhelming to patients and families. It can bring on a mix of emotions, including fear of the future, fear of dying, anxiety over family and finances, and frustration with information and treatment planning. For the patient facing a diagnosis of head and neck cancer, the reaction is intensified by the cancer site's proximity to the basic daily functions of breathing, speaking, swallowing, and eating. To better understand this, one needs only think of family gatherings or happy occasions perhaps celebrating a holiday, a birthday, or a graduation. Most people look forward to the joy of gathering with loved ones. In fact, for someone without functional limitations, these good feelings and happy memories are almost taken for granted. However, for a person with head and neck cancer, such circumstances may be approached with trepidation along with fear, anxiety, and possibly sadness. Social and family events usually include both food and conversation, activities that can be impacted by treatments for head and neck cancer. This scenario can forever change the social landscape for patients and their families.

Why does this happen? Even when head and neck cancer is treated successfully, short- and long-term quality of life concerns can be a factor in recovery. Although head and neck cancers constitute about 4% of all cancers, these patients suffer a disproportionate degree of toxic side effects. The disease and the treatment strike primary areas of daily functioning such as eating, speaking, and breathing Moreover, the impact of treatment is visible and difficult to hide (Lydiatt, Moran, & Burke, 2009). For this reason, it is important for patients, family members, and health care professionals to understand quality of life issues and their relationship to psychosocial adjustment. In particular, patients and their caregivers should be educated about quality of life, emotional distress, and compensatory strategies. Appropriate guidance and support should be made available.

There are many ways to look at and understand quality of life. It is a complex concept containing multiple layers. These concepts may vary depending on the personal situation of the patient and/or the interpreter of the situation. Quality of life and psychosocial adjustment are interrelated but are not always equal. We assume that poor quality of life will correspond to poor adjustment. But there is a subjective component that can interfere with the balance. To better understand this relationship, one must be familiar with the definitions, with the changes through the continuum of care and survivorship, and with the strategies to maximize both.

Understanding the Meaning of "Quality of Life"

The World Health Organization defines quality of life as "a state of complete physical, mental, and social well-being, and **not merely the absence of disease or infirmity**." Modern medicine has made wondrous advances in treatment options for all cancers, including head and neck cancers. Traditionally, treatment success would be measured by tumor reduction or disease-free survival. However, advances in treatment for head and neck cancer have resulted in multiple treatment choices that have equal disease-free outcomes. Consequently, new emphasis has been placed on quality of life and psychosocial adjustment to both disease and its treatment (Terrell et al., 2004). The question is no longer, "Can this cure me?" but "Can this cure me and how will it leave me?" or "What will my life be like when I am done?" These are legitimate questions and should be part of the treatment planning. The head and neck cancer patient considers survival but also must worry about functional difficulties related to swallowing, chewing, eating, and speech; they need to worry about physical symptoms such as chronic pain or dental problems (Murphy, 2009). Ultimately, they must worry about the psychosocial stressors and adaptive challenges that may result from various treatments. These challenges can create problems on an individual level, how the person feels about his or herself. Likewise, these functional deficits can create social problems and impact how survivors relate to the world around them.

Quality of life encompasses multiple dimensions. As such, one should not only consider physical health and well-being, the areas usually stressed by physicians, but emphasis must also be placed on other key elements such as satisfaction with home life, family, religion, education and/or income, ability to work, and with daily functional activities, such as eating and speaking. Yet, measuring these areas is difficult because they can be based on a subjective perception of satisfaction.

Whether you are a health care provider, a cancer patient and survivor, or the friend or family of a survivor, you likely have been in a situation where there are different points of view with regard to how a person is doing. Often, how the patient perceives quality of life may be different from how family and friends perceive it, and this may be different from the perception of the health care provider (List et al., 1999). To further compli-cate the picture, we add the dimension of how "others," that is, the community, interpret the patient's quality of life.

There is an interesting quote from a British surgeon which depicts this phenomenon: "It is hard properly to evaluate human suffering: the blind say they would rather be blind than deaf; whereas the patient without a voice considers himself fortunate that he is neither blind nor deaf" (Mehanna, 2006). Similarly, a head and neck cancer patient who has had several disfiguring surgeries but never needed radiation treatments boasts to a group of survivors, that she feels lucky that she does not have to deal with dry mouth.

This is why we are confronted with a discrepancy where a patient may report feeling fine, but family may feel that he or she is not eating enough or trying hard enough. This is also why a physician may pronounce that a patient is doing well, whereas the patient may say that he or she is "a mess." A patient may feel too embarrassed to go out with friends, whereas friends are proud of the strength and courage of the patient and want to make social plans. Understanding and interpreting quality of life is indeed a complex process. And yet it is important for patients and their loves ones to understand the basic challenges confronted during treatment and recovery from head and neck cancer and their impact on quality of life and psychosocial adjustment. Knowing what to expect can ease the potential for stress and anxiety if or when those eventualities arise. And when there is stress and anxiety, supportive services and appropriate interventions should be available to facilitate the journey of each patient and their loved ones.

To simplify the process of understanding psychosocial adjustment and quality of life, it can be helpful to view these concepts through the continuum of care, from diagnosis through survivorship. Specifically, four stages are explored: diagnosis, treatment, recovery, and long-term survivorship. The specific challenges and responses of each phase are described, along with possible interventions. Circumstances unique to new and growing patient subgroups, the HPV-related and the older patient, also are described. The ability to manage the challenges of each phase or subgroup will impact quality of life and adjustment and will lead to successful survivorship.

Diagnosis

The first stage for any cancer patient is the diagnostic stage. In the case of head and neck cancer, this involves a complex myriad of appointments and specialists, a potentially prolonged interval between the onset of symptoms and actual diagnosis and treatment planning, conflicting and sometimes unsubstantiated information complicated by the World Wide Web, and the prospect of an uncertain future. The result can be depression, frustration, anxiety, annoyance, confusion, and fear. Dealing with these issues is often difficult and may be different for each individual. This is because each patient brings unique life experiences and prior life problems to the table when confronting his or her diagnosis.

Many head and neck cancer patients bring premorbid mental health problems, such as depression, anxiety, alcohol or tobacco abuse, or cognitive decline related to age and /or addiction. It has been noted that a higher incidence of depression and even suicide exists in patients with head and neck cancer, as compared to the general cancer population (Zeller, 2006). One study examined depression among potential head and neck cancer patients. While waiting for biopsy results in a physician's office, each was given a depression survey to complete. The findings showed that those having positive biopsy results had a higher incidence of prediagnosis depression that is unrelated to their cancer (Davies, Davies & Delpo, 1986). We also know that the head and neck cancer risk factors of alcohol and tobacco abuse may lead to addiction issues and the serious problems that accompany these addictions thereby complicating treatment and recovery (Duffy et al., 2007).

It is at this moment of diagnosis that patients must confront their past history of either psychiatric or emotional problems or substance abuse. Patients with significant mental health problems may need to be assessed prior to start of treatment to enable them to manage the challenges ahead. Tobacco and alcohol abuse also must be addressed at this time. Resources for tobacco cessation programs and alcohol rehabilitative programs should be offered and education on the risks of continued use must begin. The challenge in dealing with these issues at the time of diagnosis is that patients and families primarily are concerned with the cancer. Moreover, it is an extremely stressful time for these patients and it can be more difficult to give up dependencies at times of stress. However, these topics must be put forth early and reinforced regularly as treatment begins.

Patients with head and neck cancer may also present without or with inadequate family, social, financial, or health insurance support, all factors having the potential to impact adjustment and quality of life (Rapoport, Kreitler, Chaitchik, Algor, & Weissler, 1993). Thus, it is vital for the health care team to complete a psychosocial assessment, and for the patient and family to be open and honest about their situation. Patients and their loved ones often find themselves anxious and overwhelmed in the physician's office without anyone addressing the emotional aspects of the diagnostic stage. Premorbid psychosocial problems should be addressed early with appropriate referrals followed by ongoing support. This can enhance adjustment and successful management of these aggressive treatment choices.

Quality of Life During the Treatment Stage

Once the diagnosis is made and a treatment plan is developed, the patient enters the treatment phase, bringing the often unresolved emotions and fears. At that point, patients may need to deal with the disfigurement and dysfunction that can be related to a surgical treatment. A patient may have a tracheostomy or feeding tube or may have lost his or her larynx, or part of one's tongue. These are major life changes that will also require new learning regarding self-care, speaking, or swallowing. Surgery is often followed by adjuvant chemotherapy and radiation therapy. These treatments are accompanied by pain, loss of taste, mucositis, difficulty swallowing, nausea, fatigue, and other troublesome side effects. Concurrent chemotherapy and radiation therapy may also be used as the primary treatment. This option is increasing in incidence because it allows organ preservation with avoidance of major disfiguring surgery. The cost for these gains, however, is even greater toxicities and intensified physical complaints. (Murphy, 2009) These symptoms can contribute to further emotional responses such as anxiety, irritability, frustration, disgust, depression, anger, and family strain (Sherman, Simonton, Adams, Vural, & Hanna, 2000). This phase can be very trying to the family and larger support network because of feelings of helplessness as well as individual emotional reactions (Ross, Mosher, Ronis-Tobin, Hermele, & Ostroff, 2010).

As the treatment phase begins, patients and their families need to establish new routines and incorporate the disease with day-to-day living. Multiple medical appointments, extended hospital stays and/or chemotherapy and daily radiation treatments takeover but ordinary responsibilities do not disappear and somehow patient and family need to make it work. The patient has to worry about his or her job and whether there are sick leave or short-term disability benefits. There may be a drop in income, which can cause financial strains. And the worry about health care benefits and coverage for expensive treatments and medicines is always there. Spouses or other family members worry about being there for their loved one, but also not losing their jobs at a time that finances are stressed. There may be family leave and insurance forms to be filled out: important details but extremely bothersome when all one wants to do is concentrate on treatment and cure. For the self-employed, the thought of missing work for an extended period of time creates worry about the viability of one's business and the potential for income loss. These are real fears and greatly impact adjustment as well as physical and emotional reactions to treatment.

Interventions to assist during the treatment phase include psychoeducation, information, referrals to helpful resources, and medications for pain, anxiety, and depression, as well as assistance with basic problem solving, and some simple TLC. At times, patients need only the simplest of help: someone to be there, hold a hand, and validate their feelings. Spouses and other family members need support as well as they deal with their own emotional response along with perhaps a sense of inadequacy for taking care of their loved one. Teaching relaxation exercises can provide a tool for patients and their families to take control for managing their emotions. Support groups can also be helpful, although some patients may not feel physically well enough to attend groups during treatment. Talking to a patient mentor, someone who has successfully completed similar treatment, can provide immense encouragement, especially during the rough times during treatment. Families may find it helpful to use one of the several online tools for sharing communication and organizing volunteers wanting to provide practical assistance. A few examples of these tools include, myLifeline.org (http://www.mylifeline.org), which is specifically designed for people with cancer diagnoses, CarePages (http://www.carepages.com), and Lotsa Helping Hands (http://www.lotsahelpinghands.org) and Support for People with Oral and Head and Neck Cancer (http://www.spohnc.org).

Patients, families, and members of the health care team express joy and satisfaction when treatment comes to an end. However, the toxic effects do not cease immediately following the end of treatment, and patients should be prepared for this reality. Even when patients are advised and counseled about the early and late effects of treatment, especially with combined chemotherapy and radiation treatment protocols, they often become distressed that recovery is not immediate following the conclusion of treatment, or not quick in terms of a return to normal. They are discouraged to realize that there may be chronic side effects. For some, there is suddenly a loss of the attention and activity that is found in the active treatment phase, with daily treatments and/or multiple appointments and frequent encounters with various members of the health care team (Sherman et al., 2000). There is a void of attention but toxic side effects remain strong. Signs of depression may appear at this time, even as the physical symptoms and anxiety improve. It is important to be cognizant of this potential and open to identifying signs of depression so that help may be sought in a timely fashion (Elani & Allison, 2010). It is after treatment ends that new signs of depression may develop.

Quality of Life During Recovery

Patients often get lost to follow-up during the extended recovery stage. Those with premorbid addictions and other emotional problems are especially vulnerable during this time (Duffy et al., 2009). It thus is important to reach out to these patients, to review their physical and emotional well-being, and to offer proper assistance if and when needed. Ideally, patients and families should be educated about recovery and be prepared for this stage. The National Cancer Institute has two helpful booklets in their *Facing Forward* series: "Life After Cancer Treatment," for the patient, and "When Someone You Love Has Completed Treatment," for family. These booklets provide an excellent guide during recovery on long-term survivorship. Direct interventions at this time may include referrals for rehabilitative services, such as speech and swallowing therapy, lymphedema or physical therapy, nutrition services, support groups, individual counseling, reinforcement of information about late effects of treatment, and continued follow-up with the team. This is also the time to revisit smoking and alcohol abuse where appropriate, to offer referrals for substance abuse treatment and smoking cessation. It is imperative to reinforce the risk of continued use and to support the need to successfully kick these habits.

Quality of Life and Long-Term Survivorship

Following recovery, the patient must begin to deal with the day-to-day issues related to long-term survivorship, or in simple terms, the return to normal living. Here, too, there are several phases that may be confronted during survivorship: re-integration into normal life activities, adaptation to a "new normal," and dealing with fear of recurrence, actual recurrence or metastasis, and terminal care.

The survivor re-integrates to normal life activities through actions such as returning to a regular work schedule, enjoying family and social events, participating in physical activity and exercise schedules, and again enjoying events that include food. As patients are reintegrated, there needs to be acknowledgment and acceptance that there is a "new normal." They may need to adapt to new dietary and swallowing needs, a new appearance, and to maintain alcohol and tobacco cessation. As with all cancer survivors, the fear of recurrence is omnipresent. This usually presents as anxiety with each follow-up appointment as patients focus on physical symptoms and the anxieties of family and loved ones. Support groups can be very helpful at this point. Some patients may need individual counseling if their anxieties interfere with daily functioning.

Some survivors may ultimately have to face recurrent or metastatic disease. At that time, new choices and decisions are confronted as treatment options are explored (Goldstein, Genden, & Morrison, 2008). Often, there may be discord between the family's wishes and the patient's wishes. The second time around, it can be more difficult to be positive, and the overall picture is often overshadowed by the larger unanswerable question of "Why?" There are now many more choices for treatment of advanced recurrent or metastatic head and neck cancer, and these choices are continually increasing. However, patients with head and neck cancer must consider the impact of their disease on speaking and swallowing, which will ultimately affect their quality of life. With the progression of illness, the fear of losing the ability to eat, speak, and breathe naturally grows. It is important for the health care team to acknowledge that these fears exist, to address them, and to assist with problem-solving.

In the face of advanced disease, end-of-life issues will usually enter the picture (Goldstein et al., 2008). For many, the search for ongoing treatment continues relentlessly, even as the body weakens. The question of when to stop is always present. Some patients and families report that deciding to stop treatment is a much more difficult decision than deciding what type of primary or secondary treatment to receive. The treatment team needs to ensure that they are providing adequate information to allow fully informed decisions regarding the choice of palliative care and hospice. At the same time, it is important to be cognizant of the patient and/or family's emotional state and their readiness for this discussion. This can be a difficult balance. However, the medical team needs to be compassionate and honest, so that patients and families are allowed the opportunity to understand their reality and make appropriate decisions. For head and neck cancer patients, this stage may also include critical decisions about airway management and nutrition, which can cause tension and controversy with patient, family, and healthcare professionals. Discussions regarding a tracheotomy or a feeding tube at end of life may come up. These decisions can greatly impact quality of life and should not be made lightly at a time when comfort care is the goal.

Quality of Life for Special Population Groups

The traditional risk group for head and neck cancer is middle-aged men who have abused tobacco and alcohol. However, new demographics are changing the face of head and neck cancer. New attention is being made to a unique group of HPV-related oropharyngeal cancers, primarily in the tonsil and base of tongue. The incidence of these cancers has been rising and the characteristics of this group are very different. Patients with HPV-related head and neck cancers tend to be younger men, higher socioeconomic status, and with little or no smoking or alcohol history (Maurer, D'Souza, Westra, & Forastiere., 2010). Although many of the quality of life issues related to actual treatment and side effects are similar for all subgroups, patients with an HPV-related diagnosis, have particular issues. Initially, the patient and their spouse/partner may have to deal with their reaction to the likely shock of learning that their cancer is sexually transmitted. There can be guilt, shame, and fear, which need to be dealt with through reassurance and education. On a more practical level, the average younger age of this cohort means they will have younger children. Thus, there will be a need to address the children's reactions to their parent's cancer, and to help the family best manage this. Special children's programs are offered at some cancer centers of cancer support programs, which can be helpful to younger children and to teens. There is also considerable information and support available on line by excellent groups such as Kids Konnected (http://www.kid konnected.org) and Cancer Care (http://www.cancercare.org). The National Cancer Institute also has a specific booklet geared toward teenagers, "When Your Parent Has Cancer, A Guide for Teens," (cancer.gov/1-800-4-cancer) that is beneficial for all teenagers of cancer patients. Beyond the children, the healthy spouse has to worry about family responsibilities, including those usually performed by the patient, while being a support to the family and dealing with personal emotions. The patient, who normally may be the one in charge, is now put in a needy and dependent role and must make an adaptation. There can also be concerns about job security and the possibility of being unable to maintain financial responsibilities and one's usual standard of living. Moreover, a younger age at diagnosis will usually correlate with longer survivorship and as such the late and chronic effects of treatment will have a significant role in quality of life for many years.

Another patient group of head and neck cancer patients which does not get a great deal of attention, but which is clearly increasing, is the old and "very old" segment, in particular those over the age of 80. As the general population ages, there will be higher incidence of cancers in these groups, including head and neck cancers. This group cohort faces challenges that will directly impact their quality of life due to the mere fact that a change in functional status can make the difference between independence and dependence. With age, there is the potential for greater and more serious comorbidities, which can affect treatment tolerance and survival. There also may be diminished physiologic or functional reserve, which will have a negative impact on managing the challenges of treatment. Older patients may be at greater risk for complications and toxicities that are associated with the more aggressive multimodality regimens now common to head and neck cancer (Murphy & Bond, 2008). Elderly patients and their caregivers will have more difficulty managing feeding tubes, tracheotomies, or postlaryngectomy care should they be required. There is clearly a greater caregiver burden; yet, that caregiver may be a frail spouse or a child caught in the sandwich generation. An elderly person just managing at home independently when faced with complications from major head and neck surgery or chemo/radiotherapy protocols may find him- or herself no longer able to manage at home. A supervised residential setting like assisted living or nursing homes may need to be considered, often to the dissatisfaction of the patient. Even the "fit" elderly who undergo aggressive treatments may find that it is more than their older bodies can manage and unwelcome lifestyle changes may be forced on them.

Conclusion

It is clear that quality of life factors play an important role in the survivorship experience of head and neck cancer patients. From the moment of diagnosis and on through treatment, recovery, and long-term survivorship, the physical, emotional, spiritual, and social impacts of the disease and treatment are crucial aspects of overall health outcomes. In the face of new and diverse treatment choices, often with equal outcomes, evaluating the impact of treatment on quality of life is vital. Moreover, it is imperative to identify these areas and to provide appropriate support services. When patients and caregivers understand the issues involved and are offered services that facilitate coping with their problems, they will be best able to handle their difficulties.

Ideally, cancer centers should offer appropriate support services. In the absence of this, patients and their caregivers should advocate for themselves and ask for help.

Oncology social workers are uniquely qualified to provide psychosocial support. They view the patient as part of the many systems that define their lives such as self, home, work, spirituality, financial situation, and friendships. Quality of life incorporates each of these systems so that when there is dysfunction in any of these, as has been described in this chapter, it becomes more difficult to handle the challenges of cancer. For head and neck cancer patients, with their unique concerns about basic daily functions and their high potential for emotional distress, the inclusion of psychosocial support services should be an integral part of their treatment experience. It is possible to facilitate healthy adjustment in spite of the many challenges. When the acute phase of treatment ends, it is important to provide resources to ensure successful survivorship.

References

Anderson, C., & Franke, K. A. (2002). Psychological and psychosocial implications of head and neck cancer. *Internet Journal of Mental Health*, *1*(2), 103–112.

Davies, A. D. M., Davies, C., & Delpo, M. C. (1986). Depression and anxiety in patients undergoing diagnostic investigations for head and neck cancers. *British Journal of Psychiatry*, *149*, 491–493.

Duffy, S. A., & Ronis, D. L., (2007). Depressive symptoms, smoking, drinking, and quality of life among head and neck cancer patients. *Psychosomatic*, *48*, 142–148.

Duffy, S. A., Ronis, D. L., Valenstein, M., Fowler K. E., Lambert, M. T., Bishop, C., & Terrell, J. E. (2009). Pretreatment health behaviors predict survival among patients with head and neck squamous cell carcinoma. *Journal of Clinical Oncology*, *27*(12), 1969–1975.

Elani, H. W., & Allison, P. J. (2010). Coping and psychological distress among head and neck cancer patients. *Support Care Cancer*. DOI: 10.1007/s00520-010-1013-8

El-Deiry, M., Funk, G., Nalwa, S., Karnell, L., Smith, R., Buatti, J., . . . Yao, M. (2005). Long-term quality of life for surgical and nonsurgical treatment of head and neck cancer. *Archives Otolaryngology-Head and Neck Surgery, 131*, 879–885.

Goldstein, N., Genden, E., & Morrison, S. (2008). Palliative care for patients in head and neck cancer, "I Would Like a Quick Return to a Normal Lifestyle." *Journal of the American Medical Association, 299*(15), 1818–1825.

Kohda, R., Otsubo, T. Kuwakado, Y., Tanaka, K., Kitahara, T., Yoshimura, K., & Mimura, M. (2005). Prospective studies on mental status and quality of life in patients with head and neck cancer treated by radiation. *Psycho-Oncology, 14*, 331–336.

List, M., Siston, A., Haraf, D., Schumm, P., Kies, M., Stenson, K., & Vokes, E. E. (1999). Quality of life and performance in advanced head and neck cancer patients on concomitant chemoradiotherapy: A prospective examination. *Journal of Clinical Oncology, 17*(3), 1020–1028.

Lydiatt, W. M., Moran, J., & Burke, W. J. (2009). A review of depression in the head and neck cancer patient. *Clinical Advances in Hematology and Oncology, 7*(6), 397–403.

Maurer, S., D'Souza, G., Westra, W. H., & Forastiere, A. A. (2010). HPV-associated head and neck cancer: A virus-related cancer epidemic. *Lancet, 11*, 781–789.

McCaffrey, J. C., Weitzner, M., Kamboukas, D., Haselhuhn, G., Lamonde, L., & Booth-Jones, M. (2007). Alcoholism, depression, and cognition in head and neck cancer: A pilot study. *Otolaryngology-Head and Neck Surgery, 136*, 92–97.

Mehanna, H. (2006). *History and evolution of quality of life in head and neck cancer.* Presentation at the 5th International HQROL Workshop in Head & Neck Cancer. Liverpool, U.K.

Murphy, B. (2009). Advances in quality of life and symptom management for head and neck cancer patients. *Current Opinion in Oncology, 21*, 242–247.

Murphy, B., & Bond, S. (2008). The older head and neck cancer patient. In S. Lichtman (Ed.), *Chemotherapy toxicity: Focus on the older cancer patient* (pp. 63–86). Available from: UCMPMedica, cancernetwork .com/cme .

Rapoport, Y., Kreitler, S., Chaitchik, S., Algor, R., & Weissler, K. (1993). Psychosocial problems in head-and-neck cancer patients and their change with time since diagnosis. *Annals of Oncology, 4*, 69–73.

Ross, S., Mosher, C. E., Ronis-Tobin, V., Hermele, S., & Ostroff, J. S. (2010). Psychosocial adjustment of family caregivers of head and neck cancer survivors. *Support Care Cancer, 18*, 171–178.

Sherman, A. C., Simonton, S., Adams, D. C., Vural, E., & Hanna, E. (2000). Coping with head and neck cancer during different phases of treatment. *Head and Neck, 22,* 787–793.

Terrell, J., Ronis, D. L., Fowler, K. E., Bradford, C. R., Chepeha, D. B., Prince, M. E., . . . Duffy, S. A. (2004). Clinical predictors of quality of life in patients with head and neck cancer. *Archives of Otolaryngology-Head and Neck Surgery, 130,* 401–408.

Zeller, J. (2006). High suicide risk found for patients with head and neck cancer. *Journal of the American Medical Association, 296*(14), 1716–1717.

11

MEETING THE CHALLENGES OF THE PSYCHOLOGICAL EFFECTS OF HEAD AND NECK CANCER

Sandy Cavell, MA, MSc, PGDipSci, PGDip HealthPsych
Randall P. Morton, MD

Introduction

The impact of psychological factors on head and neck patients has not been fully recognized until recently. It is now being appreciated that head and neck cancer patients can experience psychological problems not only in dealing with the disease itself but also from the adverse effects of treatment, which can not only leave patients with functional deficits affecting the ability to chew, talk, eat, swallow and restrict shoulder movement but also cause disfigurement. Head and neck cancer patients may also have to cope with ongoing physical pain.

Head and neck cancer could be described as a traumatic type of illness. In this chapter, some of the main psychological factors that are associated with head and neck cancer are discussed including mood (depression and anxiety), coping strategies, cognitive processes, quality of life, personality traits, fear of cancer recurrence, self-efficacy, and psychosocial factors. The emerging importance of the role of the psychologist in the multidisciplinary team working with the head and neck cancer patient and families, is also discussed.

Depression and Anxiety

High rates of depression and anxiety have been reported in head and neck cancer patients. In a follow-up study of head and neck cancer patients 6 months after surgery, patients reported higher levels of psychological distress than the effects of the physical impact of the disease. Despite these high levels of psychological distress, depression in head and neck patients is often underdiagnosed and not treated. Inadequate management of depression can potentially lower quality of life and may affect survival time for cancer patients.

Another study of male patients, 6 years after treatment for head and neck cancer, found a 40% rate of depression (Morton,

Davies, Baker, Baker, & Stell, 1984). This rate was confirmed in a later study. Despite that finding, depressive symptoms tend to decrease with time since treatment. Anxiety levels are often highest around the time of diagnosis and depression levels highest during treatment. De Leeuw et al. (2000), in a series of prospective studies with head and neck cancer patients, have shown that physical symptoms, depressive symptoms, levels of support, social networks, and avoidance coping can affect the risk of depression after treatment.

Depression does not appear to be directly related to physical health factors, but rather with patients' perception of the seriousness of their situation and the extent of the disruption in their lives. Depression actually correlates more closely with anxiety levels and coping strategies than the extent of treatment (Langius & Lind, 1995). Although, in very advanced disease there can be a stronger association between depression rates and physical health indicators.

Problem drinking and heavy smoking are two prevalent risk factors for the development of head and neck cancer. These risk factors can also predispose patients to depression. If the patient also believes that his or her drinking or smoking behavior caused the cancer, and if they do not give up these behaviors, this can further increase depression and anxiety levels. Continuing to smoke and drink alcohol can increase health risks and the risk of recurrence of the head and neck cancer as well as having a negative effect on quality of life (Duffy, Terrell, Valenstein, Ronis, & Copeland, 2002). The psychological effects of cancer can also impact directly on body physiology.

Immunologic Effects

Cancer research has shown that there is a relationship between immunologic competence and levels of stress, and the degree of depression and anxiety in cancer patients. Higher stress levels can cause a lowering in white blood cell counts and lessen the number of natural killer (NK) cells available to fight tumors. Increased levels of certain cytokines from immune system cells (lymphocytes) have been linked to a higher probability of metastasis in cancer. Psychological interventions that focus on reducing the arousal of the sympathetic nervous system, involving the fight-flight response can promote improved healing and faster recovery (Broadbent, Petrie, Alley, & Booth, 2001). Diaphragmatic breathing and different relaxation techniques can also reduce muscular tension, improve pain management, and lessen psychological distress.

Prognosis and Survival

There is some evidence that psychological factors can affect the progression of cancer and survival times with depression being shown to be a risk factor for overall mortality in cancer patients. Cancer patients who develop depression symptoms are two to six times more likely to die from cancer in the first 19 months compared to those without depression. Often, it is not just the length of survival but the quality of life that is important to patients.

Quality of Life

Quality of life is a subjective multidimensional phenomenon involving a perceived discrepancy between the reality of what one has and what one wants or expects (Morton, 1995). This perceived gap between reality and expectations can be shown in a quality of life measure where the individual assesses the relative importance of this "gap." A high quality of life as defined by the World Health Organization (WHO) is "a state of complete physical, mental and social well-being and not merely the absence of disease or infirmity." Much research has been done in this area with the continuing challenge being to accommodate quality of life factors into discussions of treatment options between patients and health professionals.

Often, patients with many physical symptoms and significant physical dysfunction still report high levels of life satisfaction. Associations have been found between quality of life scores and diagnosis, type and site of tumor, disease stage, and timing of testing. The site of the tumor can affect specific functions and aggregate quality of life scores. A further study found that quality of life scores improved after treatment for all stages, but remained lower for more advanced tumors. Tumor size in oral cancer has been found to be a significant predictor of post-treatment quality of life after 1 year.

Studies have shown that quality of life varies over the illness course, with overall quality of life scores usually worsening during and immediately after treatment, especially with surgical interventions. A general improvement in quality of life, at 1 year after treatment generally follows with it tending to return to pre-treatment levels. In a study following patients for 10 years, the level of quality of life was lower than in the first year or two after treatment (Mehanna & Morton, 2006a). The same authors also showed that overall quality of life rating after treatment (specifically at 12 months) was shown to be independently associated with survival in head and neck cancer patients. More unmet needs identified by patients have been shown to adversely affect quality of life and is associated with increased psychological distress.

Recurrence Concerns

Head and neck cancer patients often have great concern that cancer will return in the same site or in another part of their body, with one-third of patients in a study reporting fear of recurrence, in the 6- to 8-month follow-up period. Research has shown that up to 49% of survivors of head and neck cancer have fear of recurrence after 3 years post-treatment. The fear of recurrence does not decrease over time, which contrasts with a decreasing fear of recurrence found in general cancer patients. Survivors concerned about recurrence tend to have reduced emotional and functional wellbeing and to experience more pain and lower quality of life.

Fear of recurrence does not appear to be associated with any sociodemographic factors such as age, gender, ethnicity, marital status, or education level nor most medical factors. However, cancer concern has been associated with the persistence of symptoms, such as pain. High recurrence concern can cause patients to wrongly interpret the presence of physical symptoms as evidence of the cancer returning. This can cause considerable psychological distress to patients with them becoming hypervigilant and being involved in persistent body checking and often seeing advice from medical professionals for reassurance.

Coping

Individuals use different coping strategies to deal with their cancer experience. Coping strategies involving active/engagement skills rather than avoidance and denial approaches are more effective. Coping strategies utilized by the patient to cope with head and neck cancer can affect their quality of life. More effective coping skills are associated with lower depression and anxiety rates, higher quality of life and benefit finding and better health status. Coping by denial has been shown to be a strong predictor of future health anxiety. The use of avoidant coping strategies, involving cognitive and behavioral escape are less effective and are associated with poorer quality of life.

Active coping is considered more effective as it encourages more self-efficacy and personal control. The flexibility of the coping response to adjust to different demands of situations is an important factor. More adaptive coping may have contributed to the relatively favourable quality of life reported by laryngectomy patients, two years after surgery, despite their marked functional limitations. Currently, there is no research illustrating a consistent relationship between coping style, survival time or recurrence in cancer patients.

Other psychosocial factors influence the coping skills of individuals. Research has shown that individuals cope more effectively if they have appropriate social support, are married (Mehanna, de Boer, & Morton, 2008) and have a good relationship with their medical specialist. Difficulties with finances, transportation, housing and employment can cause added stress and adversely affect psychological functioning. Cultural factors are also important in influencing patient's attitudes to illness and medical treatment.

Cognitive Factors

Research has shown that patients often develop emotional and cognitive representations of their illness (Leventhal, Diefenbach, & Leventhal, 1992). These represesentations are based on beliefs, past experiences, and cultural influences and sometimes these representations are inaccurate and can increase anxiety. Patients also have beliefs about the cause, control, timeline and consequences of their illness, which are unhelpful and can hinder effective coping strategies. The belief in extent of personal control over the illness has been found to be related to planning and active coping (Llewellyn, Weinman, & McGurk, 2007). Negative illness perceptions were related to more maladaptive coping strategies and were associated with lower health-related quality of life. Psychoeducation needs to be provided so that patients do not have unhelpful and inaccurate ideas about their illness.

Patients who believe they have some level of control over their illness have increased perception of self-efficacy and sense of coherence that increases quality of life (Mehanna & Morton, 2006b). Also, patient beliefs about the benefits and disadvantages of taking medications and having medical procedures performed can influence their compliance behaviors, for instance, if patients are concerned about becoming addicted to painkillers they may not take the prescribed dose and struggle to cope with pain levels.

The provision of sufficient, but not too much, information is an important factor and can affect the ability of an individual to cope with his or her illness. The delivery of the "bad news" of the cancer diagnosis needs to be delivered in a sensitive way, with at least some component of "positivity" regarding what can be done to treat the disease. Appropriate medical details need to be provided so that the patient can make an informed choice about different treatment options. Medical appointments can be stressful experiences with patients often being anxious about a medical diagnosis or being focused on their illness symptoms.

Personality Factors

Personality factors can play a role in adjustment to head and neck cancer. Recent research has indicated that patients with a high level of optimism at the time of diagnosis cope better with head and neck cancer. Research has focused around the adverse psychological effects of head and neck cancer. More recent research has indicated that positive psychological changes can also occur, such as benefit finding.

Benefit Finding

Benefit finding is where there are "positive changes that result from the trauma of being diagnosed with cancer." Benefit finding can involve changes in self-perception (identity), interpersonal relationships and philosophy of life or worldview. In a recent study (Cavell, 2009) we found that 90% of head and neck cancer patients reported some benefit from their cancer experience and 60% of patients indicated that they had derived a number of benefits that had improved their lives. To understand the full extent of the patient's experience, positive aspects need to be acknowledged. Psychological benefits gained from the cancer experience may promote better psychological adjustment to the ongoing stressors of coping with cancer and promote better physical health and long-term physical functioning. Further research is needed to gain a better understanding of benefit finding as this may be an important aid in disease management and be valuable in improving psychological outcomes for patients.

Research findings indicate that benefit finding is not necessarily higher in individuals who are more severely ill but appears to be more related to the extent of life disruption, with higher benefit finding being found in individuals who perceive a greater degree of threat from their illness. Benefit finding was also more likely to occur after at least 12 months after treatment, when the individual has some time to reassess his or her life priorities.

There are other positive factors associated with benefit finding: it can broaden an individual's attentional focus and promote more varied behavioral responses. Benefit finding can also provide some psychological respite and support the continued coping and replenish psychosocial resources making individuals more physiologically resilient. Benefit finding has been linked to physiological improvement and more adaptive hormonal stress responses. Previous research has shown that individuals can experience benefit finding and still experience negative psychological effects from cancer, further research is needed to show how these negative and positive psychological effects inter-relate.

Implications for Clinical Practice

The associations found between high anxiety and depression at diagnosis and the use of dysfunctional coping strategies and poor psychological functioning after treatment, points to the importance of screening and providing psychological support to patients at diagnosis and throughout the illness trajectory so that psychological problems are less likely to arise. Consideration must be given to psychological factors, not only medical factors, in the treatment of head and neck cancer. Research findings strongly support the presence of a psychologist in the multidisciplinary head and neck cancer health care team, to promote effective ongoing psychological functioning of patients with the use of psychological screening tools and provision of appropriate and timely interventions. Additionally, this input within the multidisciplinary team allows other health care professionals to appreciate the importance of psychological input and intervention.

Treatment

Psychological interventions can address patient's concerns. Cognitive behavioral therapy (CBT) or tailored stress management programs have been shown to reduce psychological distress and anxiety and increase benefit finding in cancer patients. Altering of risk behaviors, such as smoking and drinking alcohol, can reduce depression, and fear of cancer recurrence, and have a direct impact on the physical survival and well-being of patients. Provision of appropriate psychological screening and support can then be implemented as an integral part of the clinical management of the disease. If patients are more psychologically resilient, they are more likely to cope more effectively with the stressors of the illness and ongoing physical symptoms and achieve an improved quality of life.

Conclusion

It is important for patients to realize that being anxious or depressed and having difficulty coping are common psychological effects of head and neck cancer. Patients are to be encouraged to ask for help and specialized psychological support needs to be available for these patients. The psychological effects of head and neck cancer impact differently on different individuals. Psychological interventions that promote more effective coping strategies and reduce psychological distress have been shown to be beneficial, with recent research indicating that quality of life can be improved and possibly survival rates as well. The importance of the input from psychologists trained in psycho-oncology offers the unique skill set, training, and experience to develop psychological screening tools to be used at diagnosis and deliver psychological programmes that promote better physical and psychological outcomes.

References

Broadbent, E., Petrie. K., Alley, P., & Booth, R. (2001). Psychological stress impairs early wound repair following surgery. *Psychosomatic Medicine*, *65*, 865–869.

Cavell, S. F. (2009). *Benefit finding, fear of recurrence and coping in head and neck cancer patients.* Unpublished Master's Thesis, University of Auckland, New Zealand.

De Leeuw, J. R. J., De Graeff, A., Wynand, J. G. R., Blijham, G., Hordijk, G., & Winnubst, J. A. M. (2000). Prediction of depressive symptomatology after treatment of head and neck cancer: The influence of pre-treatment physical and depressive symptoms, coping and social support. *Head and Neck*, *88*, 799–807.

Duffy, S. A., Terrell, J. E., Valenstein, M., Ronis, D. I., & Copeland, L. A. (2002). Effect of smoking, alcohol and depression on the quality of life of head and neck cancer patients. *General Hospital Psychiatry*, *24*, 140–147.

Langius, A., & Lind, M. G. (1995). Well-being and coping in oral and pharyngeal cancer patients. *Oral Oncology*, *31B*(4), 242–249.

Leventhal, H., Diefenbach, M., & Leventhal, E. A. (1992). Illness cognition: Using common sense to understand treatment adherence and affect cognition interactions. *Cognitive Theory and Research*, *16*, 143–163.

Llewellyn, C. D., Weinman, J., & McGurk, M. (2007). A cross-sectional comparison study of cognitive and emotional wellbeing in oral cancer patients. *Oral Oncology*, *44*, 124–132.

Mehanna, H. M., de Boer, M. F., & Morton, R. P. (2008). The association of psycho-social factors and survival in head and neck cancer. *Clinical Otolaryngology*, *33*(2), 83–89.

Mehanna, H. M., & Morton, R. P. (2006a). Deterioration in quality-of-life of late (10-year) survivors of head and neck cancer. *Clinical Otolaryngology*, *31*(3), 204–211.

Mehanna, H. M., & Morton, R. P. (2006b). Does quality of life predict long term survival in patients with head and neck cancer? *Archives of Otolaryngology-Head and Neck Surgery*, *132*, 27–31.

Morton, R. P. (1995). Life satisfaction in patients with head and neck cancer. *Clinical Otolaryngology and Allied Sciences, 20,* 499–503.

Morton, R. P., Davies, C., Baker, J., Baker, G., & Stell, P. (1984). Quality of life in treated head and neck cancer patients: A preliminary report. *Clinical Otolaryngology, 9,* 181–185.

12

MEETING THE CHALLENGES OF COMMUNICATION AND SWALLOWING DISORDERS AFTER TREATMENT FOR HEAD AND NECK CANCER

Bonnie Martin-Harris, PhD, CCC-SLP, BRS-S
Julie Blair, MA, CCC-SLP
Kendrea L. Focht, CScD, CCC-SLP

The processes of speaking and swallowing require little thought or effort for most healthy adults. However, the underlying complexities of these processes become evident following treatments for head and neck cancer that often involve structural and functional alterations to the mouth, throat, and esophagus. Much of what has been learned about speech and swallowing function, disorders, and treatments stems from clinical and research experiences gained from working with patients who have undergone cancer treatments to the head and neck. Although cancer treatments and rehabilitation efforts have undergone marked advances, persistent speech and swallowing dysfunction of varying degrees of severity continues to be a major problem for many survivors of head and neck cancer.

Communication

Verbal communication (speech) is reliant on the coordination of multiple interdependent subsystems. These include respiration (breathing), phonation (voicing), resonance (timbre), and articulation (forming sounds for speech). Disruption of any one of these subsystems related to a disease process, surgical alteration, or other intervention may result in altered verbal communication ability (Casper & Colton, 1998; Sullivan & Guilford, 1999; Ward & van As-Brooks, 2007).

Respiration is the driving force behind voice production. Respiratory function for voice and speech production may be impaired in a variety of ways. Patients with head and neck cancer may have a coexisting pulmonary disease, such as emphysema or chronic obstructive pulmonary disease (COPD), which increases the respiratory effort associated with talking. Respiration for speech production is also disrupted by the presence of a tracheostomy tube as most, if not all, of the lung output is redirected from the larynx (voice box) to the front of the neck out through the tracheostomy tube to ease patients' breathing. The airflow is redirected out through the tracheostomy tube; therefore, the vocal folds cannot vibrate as efficiently without the full force of airflow from below, and a breathy, weak, and/or hoarse voice typically results. Special tracheostomy valves may be placed over the opening of the tube to assist patients with directing lung air back through the larynx, thereby improving the quality and volume of the voice (Dikeman & Kazandjian, 2003; Stemple, Glaze, & Gerderman, 2000; Sullivan & Guilford, 1999; Ward & van As-Brooks, 2007).

Phonation is the process of voice production that relies on vibration of the vocal folds (vocal cords) housed in the larynx. Voice quality, pitch, and loudness (intensity) may be altered if the cancer surgery and/or radiation treatment involves the larynx or if the patient has a swallowing problem and is unable to sufficiently clear the throat after each swallow. An alternative sound source, such as an artificial larynx or special speaking valve, may be recommended in some cases when removal of the larynx is required (Casper & Colton, 1998; Stemple, Glaze, & Gerderman, 2000; Sullivan & Guilford, 1999; Ward & van As-Brooks, 2007).

Resonance is the effect on the voice related to the shape of the throat, mouth, and nasal cavities. This shaping of the sound gives rise to the timbre and richness of sound produced by the larynx. Alterations made to the shape or contours of the vocal tract following surgery to the head and neck may result in changes to the patient's and listener's perception of the voice (Casper & Colton, 1998; Stemple, Glaze, & Gerderman, 2000).

Articulation is the process through which sounds are formed by contact of the articulators, which include the tongue, jaw, teeth, palate, and lips. Approximation or full contact of these structures with one another results in the characteristic sounds used during speech production. Each sound is defined by its manner and placement. Manner refers to how the sound and airstream are shaped. Some sounds stop the flow of air, releasing it in a burst ("t"), whereas others shape the sound into a directed stream ("s"). Placement refers to where the sound is made. For example, sound can be made between the lips ("p"), tongue between the teeth ("th"), or tongue to palate ("k").

Alterations to the structure or mobility of the articulators will disrupt the precision (accuracy) of how sounds are produced. Restricted movement of the lower jaw (mandible) occurs in some patients following surgery and/or radiation treatment to the oral cavity. This condition is referred to as *trismus*, and it may interfere with articulation and resonance, as well as mouth opening for efficient eating and drinking (Casper & Colton, 1998; Sullivan & Guilford, 1999; Ward & van As-Brooks, 2007).

Treatment of the head and neck cancer through radiation, chemotherapy, and/or surgery may result in altered integrity, shape, and mobility of the structures involved in speech and voice production. In addition to influencing verbal communication ability, these changes may also have a negative impact on swallowing function (Logemann, 1998; Sullivan & Guilford, 1999; Ward & van As-Brooks, 2007).

Swallowing

Swallowing function is highly dependent on smooth and coordinated movements of the structures of the oral cavity (mouth), pharynx (throat), larynx, and esophagus (tube that moves food from the lower throat to the stomach). Swallowing is a complex process in which food and liquid are prepared in the oral cavity and transferred to the stomach. This includes mixing the food with saliva, chewing (mastication), pushing the bolus (food or liquid) through the mouth by way of upward and backward motion of the tongue, and lifting of the palate to prevent entry of the bolus into the back of the nose.

Breathing typically stops before or at least by the time the bolus reaches the back of the mouth. The bolus is then pushed through the pharynx as the larynx closes to protect the trachea (airway) and lungs from aspiration (entry of food or liquid below the vocal folds). Swallowing also includes a brisk upward and forward movement of the larynx that not only aids in closing its valves (including closing the vocal cords and the epiglottis folding over to cover the larynx), but also serves to pull open the upper part of the esophagus. There are two valves of the esophagus, one upper valve and one lower valve, which are referred to as the upper esophageal sphincter and lower esophageal sphincter, respectively. Both sphincters remain tightly closed at rest and open only to allow bolus passage during swallowing or gas, as in the case of belching (burping).

All of this dynamic activity occurs rapidly (within a couple of seconds in normal circumstances). However, following surgery, radiation, and/or chemoradiation, the structures involved in swallowing may move slower and less effectively, leading to discoordination and increased effort associated with eating and drinking (Lazarus, 2000; Murphy & Gilbert, 2009; Pauloski, Rademaker, Logemann, 1998; Sullivan & Guilford, 1999; Ward & van As-Brooks, 2007).

Swallowing Disorders

Treatment of head and neck cancer may result in a swallowing disorder (dysphagia), depending on the nature and extent of the cancer treatment. Structures and their associated function may be affected by the size and location of the tumor, and treatment modality, such as the nature of the surgical resection, type of reconstruction, and radiotherapy and/or chemotherapy treatment. For example, swallowing and speech problems after surgery are dependent on which structures were resected, the extent of resection, and sometimes, the nature of reconstruction used.

Altered sensation may interfere with airway protection if the patient is unable to feel misdirected food or liquid into the airway. Radiation and/or chemotherapy treatments may contribute to alterations in sensation and comfort during swallowing because of painful acute inflammation or swelling of the lining of the mouth and throat.

Radiation treatment may also alter the function of the salivary glands, resulting in increased thickness of secretions in the mouth and throat. Furthermore, radiation often contributes to dry mouth and throat (xerostomia), which changes the ease and pleasure associated with speaking, chewing, and swallowing. Other changes to head and neck tissues associated with radiation treatment, such as fibrosis, often result in stiffening of the mobile structures in the mouth and throat, and subsequently reduce their range of movement. Treatment involving both radiotherapy and chemotherapy may result in even more significant swallowing problems. (Lazarus, 2000; Logemann, 1998; Logemann, Pauloski, Rademaker, & Coangelo, 1997; Mittal et al., 2003; Murphy & Gilbert, 2009; Nguyen et al., 2006; Pauloski, Rademaker, Logemann, 1998; Rosenthal, Lewin, & Eisbruch, 2006; Sullivan & Guilford, 1999; Ward & van As-Brooks, 2007).

Advances in type and delivery of radiation treatment are beginning to demonstrate reduced severity of these side effects while maintaining survival rates, as well as reducing risk for long-term dysfunction after treatment is completed. The acute swallowing problems associated with head and neck treatments are usually temporary and tend to improve over time with appropriate speech and swallowing treatment. Certain medications have recently been used in an attempt to reduce the harmful effects of radiotherapy on salivary flow, which subsequently reduces severity of xerostomia. Swallowing difficulty may persist in some patients, however, long after the initial cancer treatment is completed. The nature of the swallowing treatment plan is driven by appropriate selection and implementation of standardized swallowing assessments, with unique treatment strategies specifically tailored for each individual patient (Anand et al., 2008; Logemann, 1998; Rosenthal et al., 2006; Sullivan & Guilford, 1999; Ward & van As-Brooks, 2007).

Speech and Swallowing Evaluation

Patients undergoing treatment for head and neck cancer should be seen for consultation by a speech-language pathologist whenever possible *prior* to initiation of their treatment. This initial visit is an opportunity to establish the patient's baseline communication and swallowing function, educate the patient and caregivers regarding communication and swallowing rehabilitative options following cancer treatment, and in some cases, initiate therapy prior to beginning treatment. Interaction among the head and neck cancer team is critical to maximize the recovery potential and to ensure continuity of patient care. Members of the specialty team may include some, or all of the following: otolaryngologist (ENT), nurse, speech-language pathologist (SLP), maxillofacial prosthodontist, radiologist, oncologist, gastroenterologist, dietician, physical therapist, and occupational therapist. The respective roles of each team member are detailed in other portions of this text. This specialty team creates a diagnostic and treatment plan that follows a protocol dictated not only by the cancer, but also by the nature of the speech and swallowing problems, as well as the individual needs of the patient.

There are several methods of evaluation that the clinical team may use. These tests include physical examinations and observations of movements of the mouth and throat, or evaluations that include specialized equipment for imaging and recording movements involved in voice, speech, and swallowing. These examinations are considered complementary and are often used in combination during care of patients with head and neck cancer. Tests are selected by the speech-language pathologist and physician based on the condition of the patient, clinical setting, and to answer questions regarding the patient's communication and swallowing function. It is necessary to emphasize that all of these assessment procedures require specialized training by highly skilled and competent clinicians (Carroll et al., 2007; Lazarus, 2009; Mittal et al., 2003).

Noninstrumented Evaluation

The patient and caregivers are interviewed by the speech-language pathologist as part of the initial clinical examination to gain an understanding of their perspective on their communication and swallowing ability. Voice, speech, and swallowing are often evaluated in the context of examination of the function of the structures of the face, mouth, and throat, as well as during the patient's production of sounds, words, and sentences. Swallowing observations may be made as different consistencies of liquid and textures of food are presented. The speech-language pathologist gains an impression of the patient's potential need for speech and swallowing rehabilitation throughout the examination. Clinicians are not able to precisely predict the specific nature of a patient's function prior to treatment, although they are able to gain a valuable impression of the surgical outcome based on their rehabilitative experience with other patients undergoing similar types of treatment. The speech-language pathologist is also looking for clinical signs and symptoms that may indicate a need for further instrumented speech, voice, and swallowing evaluations (Logemann, 1998).

Instrumented Examinations

The two primary instrumented examinations patients will experience involve a fiberoptic scope placed into the nose or mouth and passed to the upper throat, or radiographic imaging of the motions of swallowing. The speech-language pathologist and physician often perform both of these evaluations together although for different purposes. For example, surgeons use the examinations to assist them in diagnosing tumors and to survey structures during the post-treatment period. The speech-language pathologist, on the other hand, employs these imaging tools to determine whether and how the patient can eat and drink safely, gain knowledge of the functional outcome of the treatment, provide visual feedback to the patient during therapy, and to monitor functional changes over time. The speech-language pathologist and otolaryngologist function as a team with the patient's recovery and functional restoration as their common goal, regardless of the type of cancer treatment (Langmore, 2001; Logemann, 1998).

Communication and Swallowing Treatment

Appropriate and comprehensive speech and swallowing assessments should serve to drive the patient's treatment plan. No one treatment or management plan is appropriate for all patients, even when the patients share the same clinical circumstances regarding tumor location and staging features or undergo the same treatment modality. The selection of treatment for each individual patient is based on scientific evidence that supports the nature and type of communication and swallowing problem observed during the evaluation in order to improve function. Other factors that play into the selection of appropriate treatments include nutritional status, quality of life, social and environmental circumstances of the patient, degree of patient independence, and goals of the patient and family.

Speech and voice intervention involves educating patients on the roles of the speech subsystems and teaching compensatory strategies, or engaging the patient in active speech, voice, and swallowing exercises to maximize verbal communication and swallowing ability. Instructions to optimize oral and vocal hygiene are often included as front-line methods to improve the overall comfort and effort associated with speech, voice, and swallowing. The patient may be taught methods to maximize range of motion, strength, coordination, and speed of movement of facial, pharyngeal, and laryngeal muscles. Furthermore, patients may be instructed in therapy techniques to enhance speech resonance and improve the overall quality and clarity of voice production. Initially, patients are often instructed to slow their rate of speech and "overarticulate" (exaggerate speech movements) to improve listener intelligibility. Some patients may benefit from an oral prosthetic device to replace resected structures or to improve tongue-to-palate contact. Patients with extensive laryngeal cancer may require training with an alternative communication device, such as an electrolarynx or voice prosthesis. Many patients may require temporary use of nonverbal methods of communication immediately following surgery during the initial healing process, such as writing or using picture boards. A few patients may require long-term use of augmentative devices for communication (Casper & Colton, 1998; Logemann, 1998; Lazarus, 2000; Murphy & Gilbert, 2009; Stemple et al., 2000; Sullivan & Guilford, 1999; Ward & van As-Brooks, 2007).

Intervention for swallowing deficits often includes initial modification of liquid and/or food consistency, texture, and volume since studies and rehabilitative experience have demonstrated that the swallowing mechanism can be positively influenced by these alterations. Swallowing therapy program often integrates the effective use of postural modifications to the head, neck, and body trunk during swallowing to take advantage of the alterations that gravity provides with these postures. Patients are often instructed in the use of special maneuvers to facilitate bolus flow, bolus clearance, and airway protection. Active exercises that engage contraction muscles of the tongue and throat have also been shown to effectively impact the speed and efficiency of the swallowing process in many patients. Techniques that facilitate heightened sensation in the mouth and throat may also be applied. Some patients will benefit from adaptive feeding devices and oral appliances to assist them in placement of liquid and/or food into the mouth and help transport the bolus through the mouth (Lazarus, 2000; Logemann, 1998; Martin-Harris, 1999; Sullivan & Guilford, 1999; Ward & van As-Brooks, 2007).

In summary, multiple factors influence the degree of communication and level of swallowing difficulty that a patient may experience. The location and extent of disease, the method of treatment, coexisting health issues, and motivation of the patient all impact functional outcome. Pretreatment evaluation and counseling is vital to prepare patients and their significant others for the challenges that result from head and neck cancer treatments. Appropriate and timely evaluations and early intervention are also critical factors directed toward optimizing the functional recovery of patients. Optimal recovery and maintenance of speech, voice, and swallowing function may require an ongoing lifetime effort of consciously engaging in exercises and/ or compensatory strategies. These challenges are met through patient motivation, social support, specialized multidisciplinary team management, and continued advances in the science of rehabilitative methods.

References

Anand, A. K., Chaudhoory, A. R., Shukla, A., Negi, P. S., Sinha, S. N., Babu, A. A., . . . Vaid, A. K. (2008). Favourable impact of intensity-modulated radiation therapy on chronic dysphasia in patients with head and neck cancer. *British Journal of Radiology, 81*, 865–871.

Carroll, W. R., Lecher, J. L., Canon, C. L., Bohannon, I. A., McColloch, N. L., & Magnuson, J. S. (2007). Pretreatment swallowing exercises improve swallow function after chemoradiation. *Laryngoscope, 118*, 39–43.

Casper, J. K., & Colton, R. H. (1998). *Clinical manual for laryngectomy and head/neck rehabilitation* (2nd ed.). San Diego, CA: Singular.

Dikeman, K. J., & Kazandjian, M. S. (2003). *Communication and swallowing management of tracheostomized and ventilator dependent patients* (2nd ed.). Clifton Park, NY: Thompson Delmar Learning.

Langmore, S. (2001). *Endoscopic evaluation and treatment of swallowing disorders.* New York, NY: Thieme.

Lazarus, C. L. (2000). Management of swallowing disorders in head and neck cancer patients: Optimal patterns of care. *Seminars in Speech and Language, 21*, 293–309.

Lazarus, C. L. (2009). Effects of chemoradiotherapy on voice and swallowing. *Current Opinion in Otolaryngology and Head and Neck Surgery, 17*, 172–178.

Logemann, J. A. (1998). *Evaluation and treatment of swallowing disorders.* Austin, TX: Pro-Ed.

Logemann, J. A., Pauloski, B. R., Rademaker, A.W., & Colangelo, L. A. (1997). Speech and swallowing rehabilitation for head and neck cancer patients. *Oncology (Williston Park), 11*(5), 651–656, 659; discussion 659, 663–654.

Martin-Harris, B. (1999). Treatment of dysphagia in adults: Methods and effects [Self-study video program sponsored by the American Speech-Language Hearing Association]. Produced by Rehab Training Network—Broadcast September 16, 1999.

Mittal, B. B., Pauloski, B. R., Haraf, D. J., Pelzer, H. J., Argiris, A., Vokes, E. E., . . . Logemann, J. A. (2003). Swallowing dysfunction—Preventative and rehabilitation strategies in patients with head-and-neck cancers treated with surgery, radiotherapy, and chemotherapy: A critical review. *International Journal of Radiation, Oncology, Biology, Physics, 57,* 1219–1230.

Murphy, B. A., & Gilbert, J. (2009). Dysphagia in head and neck cancer patients treated with radiation: Assessment, sequelae, and rehabilitation. *Seminars in Radiation Oncology, 19,* 35–42.

Nguyen, N. P., Moltz, C. C., Frank, C., Karlsson, U., Nguyen, P. D., Vos, P., . . . Sallah, S. (2006). Dysphagia severity following chemoradiation and postoperative radiation for head and neck cancer. *European Journal of Radiology, 59,* 453–459.

Pauloski, B. R., Rademaker, A. W., Logemann, J. A., & Colangelo, L. A. (1998). Speech and swallowing in irradiated and nonirradiated postsurgical oral cancer patients. *Otolaryngology-Head and Neck Surgery, 118*(5), 616–624.

Rosenthal, D. I., Lewin, J. S., & Eisbruch, A. (2006). Prevention and treatment of dysphagia and aspiration after chemoradiation for head and neck cancer. *Journal of Clinical Oncology, 24,* 2636–2643.

Stemple, J. C., Glaze, L., & Gerderman, B. (2000). *Clinical voice pathology: Theory and management* (2nd ed.). San Diego, CA: Singular.

Sullivan, P. A., & Guilford, A. M. (1999). *Swallowing intervention in oncology.* San Diego, CA: Singular.

Ward, E. C., & van As-Brooks, C. J. (2007). *Head and neck cancer: Treatment, rehabilitation, and outcomes.* San Diego, CA: Plural.

Resources

Locating a Speech-Language Pathologist

The American Speech-Language-Hearing Association (ASHA). (Available online at http://www.asha.org)

Specialty Board on Swallowing and Swallowing Disorders (BRS-S). (Available online at http://www.swallowingdisorders.org)

Cookbooks and Online Recipes

Achilles, E. (2004). *The dysphagia cookbook: Great tasting and nutritious recipes for people with swallowing difficulties.* Nashville, TN:

Cumberland House. A specialty cookbook filled with nutritious, great-tasting recipes. (Available online at http://www.dysphagia.com)

Clegg, H., & Miletello, G. (2001). *Eating well through cancer: Easy recipes and recommendations during and after treatment.* Memphis, TN: Favorite Recipes® Press.

Dethero, B. R. (1999). *Let's do lunch.* Cleveland, OH: Dethero Enterprises. A handbook with nonchew recipes. (Available online at http://www.dinner throughastraw.net)

Goldberg, P. Z. (1980). *So what if you can't chew, eat hearty!: Recipes and a guide for the healthy and happy eating of soft and pureed foods.* Springfield, IL: Charles C. Thomas Publisher. (Available online at http://www.amazon.com)

Katz, R. (2004). *One bite at a time: Nourishing recipes for cancer survivors and their friends.* Berkeley, CA: Celestial Arts. (Available online at http://www.amazon.com)

Nestlé Nutrition. (2011). Recipes. Web site offers Resource® ThickenUp® dysphagia recipes, included recipes for energy and recipes using fruit. (Available online at http://www.nestlenutrition.co.uk)

Richman, J. W. (1994). *Pureed foods with substance and style.* Sudbury, MA: Jones & Bartlett Publishers. (Available at http://www.amazon.com)

SPOHNC. (2005). *Eat well—stay nourished: A recipe and resource guide for coping with eating challenges.* Lenexa, KS: Cookbook Publishers. (Available online at http://www.spohnc.org)

Thigpen, P. A. (1999). *Dinner through a straw.* Cleveland, OH: Dethero Enterprises. A favorite handbook for patients of oral surgery and others who cannot chew. (Available online at http://www.dinner throughastraw.net)

Weihofen, D. L., & Marino, C. (1998). *The cancer survival cookbook: 200 quick ways with helpful eating hints.* Nourishing recipes and practical advice are provided to help cancer patients in their recovery. New York, NY: John Wiley and Sons. (Available online at http://www.amazon.com)

Weihofen, D. L., & Robbins, J. (2002). *Easy-to-swallow, easy-to-chew cookbook.* New York, NY: John Wiley and Sons. Packed with more than 150 tasty and nutritious recipes for people who have difficulty swallowing. (Available online at http://www.amazon.com)

Wilson, J. R. (2003). *The I can't chew cookbook: Delicious soft diet recipes for people with chewing, swallowing, and dry mouth disorders.* Alameda, CA: Hunter House. (Available online at http://www.amazon.com)

Wimmer Cookbooks. Collection of 200 easy recipes to help cancer patients tolerate treatment. (Available online at http://www.amazon.com)

Womack, P. (1999). *The dysphagia challenge: Techniques for the individual.* (Available online at http://www.dysphagiabooks.com)

Womack, P. (2011). Dysphagia books: resources for swallowing disorders. Web site offers online recipes and allows you to order dysphagia books. (Available online at http://www.dysphagiabooks.com)

Woodruff, S., & Gilbert-Henderson, L. (2008). *Soft foods for easier eating cookbook: Easy-to-follow recipes for people who have chewing and swallowing problems.* Garden City Park, NY: Square One Publishers. (Available online at http://www.dysphagia-diet.com/books.htm)

Wright, C. (2005). *Second helpings.* Salem, VA: Author. 75 recipes developed by a caregiver for her husband who has difficulty chewing and swallowing. (Available at: http://www.secondhelpingsbycacky.com)

Resources for Thickening Agents

Bruce Medical
411 Waverley Oaks Road, Suite 154
Waltham, MA 02452
1-(800)-225-8446 (toll free)
http://www.brucemedical.com

Diafoods: Thick-It®
Milani Foods, 800-333-0003
East of the Mississippi: Health Call at 800-778-5704
West of the Mississippi: Kansas Specialty Service
at 877-751-5095
http://www.thickitdelivered.com
http://www.walgreens.com
http://www.brucemedical.com/thickit.htm
Thickens hot, cold, and pureed foods. Pharmacies
will order for you.

Diversified Medical Equipment and Supplies, Inc.
15472 Chemical Lane
Huntington Beach, CA 92649
1-(888)-515-DMES (3637) (toll-free)
1-(714)-657-7615 (fax)
http://dmes.com

Hormel HealthLabs
http://www.dysphagia-diet.com/hhl.htm

Hydra~Aid Gel Liquid Thickener
http://www.thickitretail.com

Med-Diet
http://www.dysphagia-diet.com

Nestlé Nutrition
1-(888)-240-2713 (toll-free)
http://www.nestlenutritionstore/com

Novartis: Resource® Thickenup®
http://www.dysphagia-diet.com/novartis.htm

Nutra/Balance Company
Regular Instant Thickener
155 Wadsworth Way
Indianapolis, IN 46219
1-(800)-654-3691 or 1-(317)-356-5478
http://www.nutra-balance-products.com

WisdomKing.com, Inc.
4015 Avenida de la Plata, Unit 401
Oceanside, CA 92056
1-(877)-931-9693 (toll-free)
1-(760)-450-0675 (fax)
http://www.wisdomking.com/food-thickeners

Resources for Modified Feeding Utensils and Cups

Bruce Medical
411 Waverley Oaks Road, Suite 154
Waltham, MA 02452
1-(800)-225-8446 (toll-free)
http://www.brucemedical.com

DysphagiaPlus, LLC
7337 Capistrano Drive
Shreveport, LA 71105
1-(800)-581-8127 (office)
1-(800)-597-9839 (fax)
http://www.dysphagiaplus.com

RehabMart, LLC
150 Sagewood Drive
Winterville, GA 30683-1563
1-(800)-827-8283 (toll free)
1-(706)-213-1144 (direct)
1-(603)-843-2144 (fax)
http://www.rehabmart.com/category/Dining_Aids.htm

WisdomKing.com, Inc.
4015 Avenida de la Plata, Unit 401
Oceanside, CA 92056
1-(877)-931-9693 (toll-free)
1-(760)-450-0675 (fax)
http://www.wisdomkking.com/eating-aids

13

MEETING THE CHALLENGES OF GOOD NUTRITION

Jennifer Thompson, RD, LD, CNSD

This chapter on nutrition aims to provide useful information to patients with oral and head and neck cancer and their caregivers. Although this information may be well known to some, it may be the first time others have considered what they eat as more than something to satisfy cravings. After reading this chapter, you should be able to understand why nutrition is important and how to include it in the fight against cancer.

Good Nutrition for Oral and Head and Neck Cancer Patients

The definition of "good" nutrition varies depending on an individual's circumstances. The ideal or most beneficial dietary intake for the public is not always the best diet for those who have cancer. During cancer treatment the nutritional needs of a person are usually higher than normal. This means if someone required 2,000 calories a day before being diagnosed with cancer, the need may increase to 2,500 or 3,000 calories a day during treatment. One way to measure whether you are eating adequately is to follow your weight on a weekly basis. If your weight stays the same or is stable, then you are probably eating well enough (unless you are retaining fluid). If you start to see weight loss, then it may be time to make some changes.

Even if individuals are overweight, it is still important for them to consume adequate calories. Many people think, "I have extra weight to lose. I'll be OK." However, cancer alters the body's metabolism as do stressful situations such as undergoing chemotherapy and/or radiation therapy. Thus, muscle wasting occurs along with fat loss, leaving patients weak at a time when they need strength.

A Balanced Diet

The details of what a balanced diet looks like are listed in Table 13–1. Basically, it means eating a variety of foods every day. Nutrients are found in many different foods, yet each food

Table 13–1. 2010 USDA Daily Recommendations* for Men Ages 31 to 50

Food Group	Servings Per Day
Calories	2,200
Fruit	2 cups
Vegetables	3 cups
Grains	7 ounces
Meats/beans	6 ounces
Dairy	3 cups
Oil	6 teaspoons
"Discretionary" or free to choose	290 calories

*Released January 31, 2011 after thorough review of latest scientific research. Go to http://www.mypyramid.gov to find out your personal needs.

group also contains nutrients that are unique to that group. In addition, one group may be a better source of nutrients than another group. For example, iron found in leafy green vegetables is poorly absorbed, but iron found in red meat is an excellent source because it is absorbed very well. Therefore, any diet that requires you to eliminate a food group completely should be carefully examined. Talk to your health care provider if you are considering following a new diet or if you are having difficulty with your current diet. Your ability to eat a balanced diet in the amounts recommended may be limited, and the means by which nutrition is obtained may need to be altered. A registered dietitian (RD) is an expert in all aspects of nutrition. If your cancer center does not have an RD on staff, go to http:www.eatright.org to locate one in your area.

Why Nutrition Is Important

There is evidence that maintaining a well-nourished body helps a person handle a treatment regimen better. "Research shows that poor nutritional status and inadequate dietary intake have a negative impact on outcomes of cancer therapy, including increased risk for complications, poor tolerance, and response to treatment and a lower quality of life" (Jacobsen, 2006).

Screening Head and Neck Patients for Nutritional Risk

The following signs or symptoms place a cancer patient at risk for malnutrition:

- Weight loss (unintentional)
- Loss of appetite (referred to as anorexia in medical terms)
- Difficulty chewing or swallowing (referred to as dysphagia)
- Poor dietary intake (usually related to loss of appetite and difficulty chewing or swallowing)
- Feeling full quickly when eating (referred to as early satiety)
- Nausea, vomiting, or diarrhea that persists for more than a day or two
- Oral mucositis (inflammation of the lining of the mouth and throat) secondary to radiation therapy and chemotherapy.

Nutritional Therapy

Nutritional therapy involves using the diet to achieve a certain goal. During cancer treatment, the main goal of nutrition is to support patients so they are able to withstand the surgery, radiation, and/or chemotherapy. A poor diet can cause patients to have their cancer treatment stopped or postponed temporarily if they are too weak to handle treatment-related stress. It can also delay the healing process once the treatment is completed.

Maintaining Good Nutrition During Treatment

Attitude plays a key role in the ability to maintain good nutrition during treatment. When you are physically worn out and if you experience any of the symptoms listed previously, you may struggle with eating or drinking anything, much less everything your body needs. Your general mind-set will be important. If you believe nutrition is vital to your success during treatment, you will be more likely to make yourself do more than you thought possible. A pronutrition mindset may have other benefits, such as causing less friction or resistance when caregivers are encouraging you to eat or when health care providers are giving recommendations for using a feeding tube.

The Role of Vitamins and Minerals

Vitamins, minerals, and phytonutrients play a variety of roles in the daily functions of the body and are as necessary as carbohydrates, protein, and fat. Without adequate vitamins and minerals, the body is unable to fully utilize the calories consumed. However, high intake of vitamins and minerals can be unsafe during active treatment and is not generally recommended. Before you start your treatment, talk with your health care provider about any vitamin or mineral supplements you are already taking or considering. Some cancer centers will advise not to take any supplements, even a general multivitamin, during days of radiation or chemotherapy. Outside of radiation and chemotherapy days, a general multivitamin with minerals that contains no more than 100% RDA (recommended dietary allowance) should be sufficient.

Herbal Supplements

Talk with your health care provider *before* you start taking any herbal supplements. Many herbal supplements have interactions with medicines, including chemotherapy drugs, which may be undesirable. Additionally, herbs from foreign countries are not regulated. If your doctor is unfamiliar with the supplements you are interested in taking, the dietitian or pharmacist may be able to provide information for you on their safety during treatment. Any information you read about dietary or herbal supplements must be carefully examined. Go to http://www.quackwatch.com or http://www.mskcc.org/aboutherbs for information about these supplements.

Feeding Tubes

Your doctor may suggest that a feeding tube be put in place before you begin treatment to provide a route for water, nutrition, and medicines when you are unable to adequately consume these substances orally. A feeding tube is a necessary tool because the mouth and/or throat may become very sore during cancer treatment involving surgery, radiation, and/or chemotherapy. The length of treatment may vary, as may the time for healing, from several weeks to several months. Thus, the feeding tube provides a way for you to give your body the nourishment it needs to withstand the treatment and to recover as quickly as possible. You may use the feeding tube occasionally in the beginning, but it may eventually become the only way you are able to get water and "food." If you are still wary about its value, consider it a potential stress-reliever. With a feeding tube, you and your caregivers won't have to worry about how you are going to drink or eat when there is discomfort in your mouth and throat. There is adequate evidence in the medical literature to show that patients who are malnourished do not respond as well to chemotherapy or radiation therapy.

Supplementing the Diet to Maintain Balance

When food no longer appeals to you or when it is too painful to chew and swallow, then it is time to consider nutritional supplements. If you find yourself struggling with eating from a lack of appetite, then supplements come in handy because drinking may be an easier and quicker way to get the calories. If you start to develop sores in the mouth and throat but are still able to tolerate liquids, then supplements can provide a concentrated source of nutrition. If you find yourself unable to tolerate anything by mouth, supplements may be put into the feeding tube.

Supplements are divided into those intended to be consumed by mouth and those that are meant to be given through a feeding tube.

Oral Supplements

These supplements can be given through the feeding tube as well. Most supplements contain a combination of fat, protein, carbohydrates, vitamins, and minerals. However, there are supplements that contain only protein to help patients who are unable to meet the demands for protein because they are unable to tolerate chicken, beef, pork, fish, and seafood. The remaining discussion will focus on those supplements that contain a combination of nutrients. Table 13–2 presents specific information on current supplements available.

Clear liquid or "milky." Many people are surprised to learn that there are clear liquid supplements available. They are often described as juice-like with the added benefit of having protein added to them. The "milky" supplements are more common, but they are not all milk based. Some use soy milk instead of cow's milk. Regardless of the milk used, all supplements are lactose-free.

Powder or ready-to-drink. There are versions that come in powder form and require some liquid to make them tolerable. The ready-to-drink versions are available in cans or resealable bottles. Unopened, they can be kept at room temperature or refrigerated, but they should be kept in the refrigerator after opening.

Table 13–2. Nutritional Supplements

Nestle Products (Formerly Novartis)					
Product	**Flavors**	**Cal**	**Prot**	**Fiber**	**Admin**
Benecalorie	Unflavored	330	7 g	0	Oral
Boost	Multi	240	10 g	0	Oral
Boost Plus	Multi	360	14 g	0	Oral
Boost High Protein	Multi	240	15 g	0	Oral
Boost Glucose Control (DM)	Multi	190	16 g	3 g	Oral
Boost Hi-Protein Powder*	Van	200	13 g	0	Oral
Nutrament* (12 oz)	Multi	360	16 g	0	Oral
Resource 2.0*	Van (available in 8 oz. or 32 oz.)	475	21 g	0	Oral
Resource HealthShake*	Van	270	9 g	0	Oral
Resource Shake Plus*	Multi	480	15 g	0	Oral
Resource Boost Breeze	Orange, Peach, Wild Berry	250	9 g	0	Oral

All products are available at stores unless indicated by *; online sites include http://www.boost.com and http://www.walgreens.com; telephone numbers are 800-828-9194 (Walgreens), 800-438-6153 (TAD), and 800-446-6380 (Redline).

Table 13–2. *continued*

Nestle Products

Product	Flavors	Cal	Prot	Fiber	Admin
Carnation Instant Breakfast (CIB) powder	St, choc, van	130	5 g	0	Oral
CIB Plus	St, choc, van	375	13 g	0	Oral
CIB Very High Calorie (VHC)	Van only	560	23 g	0	Oral
Fibersource HN	Unflavored	300	13.4 g	2.5 g	Tube
Nutren	Van	250	15.6 g	3.4 g	Oral/tube

Nestle products are generally ordered online or by telephone; the CIB powder is available in stores as well. Online sites include http://www.carnationinstant breakfast.com and http://www.nestle-nutrition.com.

There are a variety of Nutren products that vary in calorie level, fiber content, and indications for use. Your dietitian can help you determine which one is right for you.

Ross Products

Product	Flavors	Cal	Prot	Fiber	Admin
Ensure	Multi	250	9 g	0	Oral
Ensure Plus	Multi	350	13 g	0	Oral
Ensure High Protein	Multi	230	12 g	0	Oral
Ensure Fiber	Van, choc	250	8.8 g	2.8 g	Oral
Ensure Pudding (8 oz)	Multi	340	8 g	2 g	Oral
Glucerna Shake (DM)	Multi	220	10 g	2.8 g	Oral
Juven*	Grape, orange	78	14 g	0	Oral

continues

Table 13–2. *continued*

Ross Products *continued*					
Product	**Flavors**	**Cal**	**Prot**	**Fiber**	**Admin**
Jevity* (also comes in variations with more calories and protein for the same volume)	Unflavored	250	10.4 g	3.4 g	Oral/tube
Osmolite* (also comes in variations with more calories and protein for the same volume)	Unflavored	250	8.8 g	0	Oral/tube
Two Cal HN*	Van, butter pecan	475	20 g	1.2 g	Oral/tube

RepleteRoss products are available at stores unless indicated by *; online sites include http://www.ross.com. Telephone number: 800-986-8502.

Scandipharm (Axcan pharma)					
Product	**Flavors**	**Cal**	**Prot**	**Fiber**	**Admin**
Scandishake (powder that is mixed with milk primarily but can also be mixed with other liquids)	Multi	600	6 g	0	Oral
Scandical (tablespoon) (powder that is added to foods to increase the calorie content)	Unflavored	35	0	0	Oral

Order from: Telephone 800-472-2634; http://www.axcan.com or store.axcanscan dipharm.com

Table 13–2. *continued*

Nutra/Balance

Product	Flavors	Cal	Prot	Fiber	Admin
Nutra/Shake 2.0	Multi	470	20 g	0	Oral
Nutra/Shake Supreme	Multi	400	12 g	0	Oral

Order from: Telephone 800-654-3691; http://www.nutra-balance-products.com

Resurgex

Product	Flavors	Cal	Prot	Fiber	Admin
Resurgex Select	Multi	350	15 g	0	Oral

Order from: Telephone 877-737-8749; http://www.resurgex.com

Protein Powder Options

Product	Flavors	Cal	Prot	Fiber	Admin
Resource Beneprotein (Novartis) 1 scoop	Unflavored	25	6 g	0	Oral
EvoPro 1 scoop (http://www.cytosport.com)	Multi	140	26 g	0	Oral
Mega-Isolate 2 scoops (GNC) http://www.gnc.com	Van, choc	230	50 g	1 g	Oral

continues

Table 13–2. *continued*

Weight Gainer Powder Options

Product	Flavors	Cal	Prot	Fiber	Admin
Weight Gainer 1850 (GNC) http://www .gnc.com 3 cups powder mixed with 3 cups 2% milk	Multi	1,850	74 g	0	Oral
Russian Bear 5000 (suggested to mix with 1 gallon of whole milk to reach 5,000 calories) http://www.nice muscle.com	Van, choc	2,600	184 g	0	Oral
Twinlab Mass Fuel (suggested to mix 4 scoops to 3 cups milk) http://www.nice muscle.com	Van, choc	600	50 g	0	Oral

Products with (DM) are lower in total carbohydrates and specifically made for people with diabetes. However, many of the other supplements can still be used by people with diabetes. A dietitian can help you determine the best fit for you. Often, the timing and amount of supplement consumed at each time can be modified to allow most of these products to be used.

Product nutrient values and ingredients are subject to change. See the product label or contact the manufacturer for the most current information.

To locate a dietitian or nutritionist, you may request a referral from your physician or contact the American Dietetic Association (http://www.eatright.org).

DISCLAIMER: Product data are provided to readers as a convenience and guide only. SPOHNC does not recommend nor endorse any product listed herein. Consult your physician prior to using any of the products mentioned.

Regular, plus, high protein. To add further to the decision-making process, you will find different names for the same basic product. The "regular" option is the base model and contains approximately 240 calories and 10 grams of protein. The "plus" option contains more calories and protein, approximately 350 calories and 13 to 15 grams of protein per serving. The "high protein" option usually keeps the calories about the same as the "regular" but adds more protein. There are even some supplements that contain 560 to 600 calories.

Brand name or generic. The common brand-name supplements that most people are familiar with are Ensure and Boost. Anybody who has tried either one will be glad to share their opinion, but try them for yourself and see which one you like best. Most people end up preferring one over the other. A few will like both and some will dislike both. Fortunately, they are not the only supplements on the market. There are other products, including generic versions that are usually more economical.

Tube Feed Supplements

One big difference between these supplements and the oral alternatives is the lack of flavor. Otherwise, these supplements are the same in content. The choices to be made among these formulas include calorie content and any special ingredients or formulations. For calories, the range is typically from 240 to 480 per can. This affects you in two ways: (a) the number of cans needed to meet your needs and (b) the amount of water provided to help with hydration. Two examples of special ingredients are fiber and omega-3 fatty acids. Some supplements contain formulas that are disease specific such as those designed for patients with renal or kidney disease.

Your dietitian can assist you in determining the best formula for you and your unique situation and may be able to provide you with samples of supplements. You can try different brands and flavors to see which ones suit you or which ones work best as a tube feeding.

Throughout this section, the who, what, when, where, and why of nutrition have been discussed so that patients and caregivers may be better equipped for their fight against cancer. A well-nourished body will be able to better withstand the surgery, radiation, and/or chemotherapy treatment. Here is a good visual comparison to help you remember the importance of nutrition: Imagine yourself as a car. No one expects a car to run on empty. It must be filled with gas on a regular basis to run effectively. Food is your fuel to keep you running well.

The information provided in this section is not all inclusive. Your local dietitian will be glad to work with you on a one-on-one basis to personalize your nutrition. You should not be hesitant to ask your doctor for a referral to a dietitian. If the facility where you are receiving treatment does not have a dietitian available, you can find one on http://www.eatright.org.

Reference

Jacobsen, M. (2006, Spring). Getting the word out: Nutrition counseling improves outcomes. *Oncology Nutrition Connection, 14*(2).

14

MEETING THE CHALLENGES OF INSURANCE ISSUES

A. HEALTH INSURANCE IN THE UNITED STATES

Beth Patterson, President, Mission Delivery
Pat Jolley, RN, BS, Chief of Patient Services
Erin Moaratty, Chief of External Communications
Tammy Neice, RN
Elaine Martinez, LPN
Tanya Walker, RN, BSN

Advances in medical technology and medicine make health insurance a necessity in the 21st century. As people are living longer, the size of the aging population is increasing, and, unfortunately, data shows that as we become more technically advanced, we are also moving away from healthier lifestyles. After years of debate, the "Patient Protection and Affordable Care Act" (PPACA) was signed into law on March 23, 2010, with the implementation of the law being phased in over multiple years. For many Americans, it's been difficult to determine how the new laws will affect them and their families. Beginning in 2010, children and young adults were provided two major coverage advances—the elimination of pre-existing condition exclusions for children under 19 and extension of dependent coverage under the parent's insurance policy for young adults under the age of 26.

Additionally, the PPACA includes the following provisions that will benefit patients in the near future: businesses with fewer than 50 employees will receive tax credits covering up to 50% of employee premiums; Community Health Centers will receive an additional $11 billion in funding to expand; health plans will be required to spend 80% of premium dollars on clinical services and quality activities in the individual and small group markets and 85% in the large group market effective January 1, 2011. Another important reform will become effective on January 1, 2014, when all insurance companies will be prohibited from denying coverage based on pre-existing conditions.

The PPACA will eliminate health care access and financial burdens faced by many patients including those with serious diagnoses such as cancer. To learn more about the health reform law and understand how it will affect you visit http://www .healthcare.gov or http://www.insureUStoday.org .

Most Americans obtain health insurance coverage through their employer as part of a group health benefit. Employer-sponsored group health plans must cover all employees regardless of their medical history. There is an open enrollment period, decided by the employer, at which time all employees who have not yet signed up for insurance have the ability to do so. The insurance carrier can impose a pre-existing condition clause on individuals who did not have previous health coverage, also known as credible coverage. The clause will exclude charges related to the pre-existing condition(s) only. This clause is typically 12 months in duration and at 12 months and 1 day the person is covered the same as any other insured employee. If an employee had coverage previously, the plan may opt to credit previous coverage instead of imposing the entire 12-month waiting period for the condition.

Most employer-sponsored group health plans are federally regulated by the Employee Retirement Income Security Act of 1974 (ERISA). ERISA outlines the process for appealing a claim. Another benefit of employer-sponsored group health plans is that insured employees can elect to continue their group coverage if they leave their employer. Federal law mandates that employers with 20 or more employees must offer COBRA, the (Consolidated Omnibus Budget Reconciliation Act). Additional information on both programs is reviewed at the end of this chapter.

If you are self-employed, check to see whether your state has any health insurance companies that offer group health plans for groups of one. Availability will vary by state, and requirements will differ by insurance company. To learn whether your state offers this coverage, contact a local insurance agent and/or the National Association for the Self-Employed (http://www.nase.org).

If you are facing the loss of your group insurance plan, an individual insurance plan may be an option, depending on your medical history. If you have a previous health condition, you may be subject to a rider that excludes coverage for any condition previously diagnosed or may enforce a pre-existing condition waiting period. The length of the waiting period must be disclosed to you if it is imposed. Individual plans are subject to state laws. The Pre-Existing Condition Insurance Plan (PCIP) was created to make health insurance available to individuals who have had a problem accessing health insurance due to an existing medical condition. States were given the option to administer PCIP themselves or to have the federal government administer it for them. The PCIP covers a wide range of health benefits, including primary and specialty care, hospital care, and prescription drugs. The plan will not charge a higher premium based on an individual's medical condition and does not base eligibility on income. Enrollees are required to be a citizen of the United States or lawfully present in the United States, be uninsured for the 6 months prior to applying and must have had a problem obtaining insurance due to a pre-existing condition. Information and applications for the PCIP can be accessed at http://www.pcip.gov .

As with auto or homeowner policies, a health insurance policy conveys that you are entering into a contract with the insurance company. Regardless of insurance carrier and type of insurance, group or individual, health maintenance organization (HMO), preferred provider organization (PPO), or a high deductible health plan (HDHP), you are subject to the terms of your policy. It is very important that you read your plan carefully. If you have questions about any portion of your policy, ask them. If you have coverage under a group health plan or individual plan, refer to the phone number provided on your insurance card. If your insurance was through your employer, you can contact your human resources department for assistance.

Network Providers and UCRs

Most health insurance policies covering Americans today use a specified "network" of providers. You generally have the best reimbursement rate when you utilize providers who participate within your insurance carrier's network. These providers may include physicians, hospitals, outpatient diagnostic facilities, radiation therapy centers, outpatient infusion centers, or any other provider of medical services, and have a contract with the insurance plan. Remaining within the provider network is the most effective way to keep your out-of-pocket expenses to a minimum.

Your insurance carrier is responsible for annually providing beneficiaries with a listing of participating providers. However, it is in your best interest to verify at the time you are scheduling an appointment that the provider is still a participating provider as provider networks change throughout the year.

When your insurance carrier receives a claim on your behalf, it processes claim payments per the terms of the contract. Once the claim has been processed, the provider and the patient both receive statements, (either electronically or written). These statements are more commonly referred to as an "explanation of benefits" (EOB). It is important to review each EOB you receive because they will tell you the amount paid to the provider as well as any financial responsibility you may have. If a discrepancy exists, this is evidence you will need to contact your insurance company and/or provider so that the error can be corrected.

Out-of-Network Providers and UCRs

You may choose to go to a provider who is not within your provider's network. *However,* before you seek care outside of your provider's network, check your insurance policy and make sure that you have out-of-network (OON) benefits. If you do not have OON benefits and you do elect to receive care at an OON facility, you may be responsible for the entire bill. If you have OON benefits, your claim will be processed using the prevailing usual, customary, and reasonable (UCR) rates for the services provided. UCR refers to the maximum amount that will be paid for services that are eligible to be reimbursed under your insurance policy. Most insurance policies only pay a percentage of what is determined to be the customary rate for your local area. For example, if your plan covers 80% of UCR charges you are responsible for the remaining 20%. In addition, the provider may "balance bill" you for the difference between what the provider charges and what the insurance company pays.

As the following example illustrates, the amount of patient financial responsibility can be much greater than originally anticipated. The application of UCR rates and balance billing can more than double the patient's financial responsibility.

In Network Example:

Doctor Visit

Actual Charge $250.00

UCR Allowable Charge $200.00

Contractual Write-Off $50.00

80/20 plan Insurance Paid . . . $160.00

Your 20% Co-Insurance $40.00

Your Total Costs $40.00

OON and UCR Example:

Doctor Visit Actual

Charge $250.00

UCR Allowable Charge $200.00

60% (OON) Insurance Paid . . . $120.00

Your 40% Co-Insurance $80.00

Balance Billing Cost OON $50.00

Your Total Costs $130.00

Even if your policy has an out-of-pocket maximum, it is important to understand that *only* your portion of the UCR allowed amount is applied toward your maximum. In the example just given, only $80 (your portion of the amount the insurance company deemed payable) of the $130 you paid would count toward your yearly out-of-pocket maximum. For this reason, many patients have much larger than anticipated medical bills when seeking services at an OON provider.

Medicare and UCRs

UCR charges are not regulated by state or federal agencies, but Medicare publishes a UCR fee schedule. This is commonly referred to as Medicare allowable charges. Providers who participate with Medicare agree to accept the Medicare allowable charge as full payment. Bear in mind that the patient will be responsible for the co-insurance and deductible.

Example:

Chemotherapy actual charge $500

UCR allowable charge $300

Medicare 80/20 insurance paid . . . $240

Your 20% coinsurance $60

Your total costs $60

Medicare providers may choose not to bill the patient for amounts above the Medicare allowable fee schedule. It is important to verify that your provider "accepts Medicare assignment" or is a "Medicare provider" to avoid unexpected and potentially large out-of-pocket expenses.

Sometimes, a health care provider will notify patients, either verbally or by written notification that they may be subject to balance billing after the insurance carrier has paid the allowable charge or if the claim is denied completely for reimbursement. This communication constitutes a "waiver of financial responsibility" and is also known as Advanced Beneficiary Notice (ABN). This happens most commonly when a health care provider anticipates that the insurance carrier may deny a claim and the physician and patient want to proceed with the therapy regardless of the insurance coverage.

All insurers, including Medicare, provide an appeal process for denial of service. To understand more about how to appeal, please refer to *Your Guide to the Appeals Process* from the Patient Advocate Foundation (PAF) or contact PAF directly at 800-532-5274.

Employee Retirement Income Security Act of 1974 (ERISA)

ERISA is a federal law that was established to protect the rights of employees and the security of their retirement funds and medical benefits provided by an employer. ERISA sets minimum standards for most voluntarily established pension and health plans in private industry to provide protection for individuals in these plans.

In general, ERISA covers any employer with a retirement plan and/or employee benefit plan. Only a few plans are exempt, such as group health plans established or maintained by governmental entities (federal, state, and local); church plans; or plans that are maintained solely to comply with applicable workers' compensation, unemployment, or disability laws. ERISA also does not cover plans maintained outside the United States primarily for the benefit of nonresident aliens or unfunded excess benefit plans. For more information about ERISA, visit http://www.dol.gov/dol/topic/health-plans/erisa.htm

Amendments to ERISA

There have been a number of amendments to ERISA, expanding protections available to health benefit plan participants and beneficiaries. One important amendment, the Consolidated Omnibus Budget Reconciliation Act (COBRA), provides some workers and their families with the right to continue their health coverage for a period of 18 months, with an extension option of an additional

11 months if deemed disabled by the Social Security Administration. Another amendment is the Health Insurance Portability and Accountability Act (HIPAA), which provides important new protections for working Americans and their families and who have group benefits and who might otherwise be uninsurable. Other important amendments include the Newborns' and Mothers' Health Protection Act, the Mental Health Parity Act, and the Women's Health and Cancer Rights Act.

Requirements of Employers

ERISA requires that sponsors of private employee benefit plans provide participants and beneficiaries with adequate information regarding their plans. In addition, under the ERISA law, your employer must provide you with a copy of your summary plan description (SPD) and plan document within 120 days after the plan becomes effective. The plan administrator must also distribute SPDs to participants and beneficiaries every 5 years unless no changes have occurred, at which time the administrator may wait 10 years. If a beneficiary requests a copy of the SPD and/ or complete plan language in writing, it must be supplied within 30 days after receiving the written request. The request must be made to the plan administrator with reference to the ERISA law. Failure to comply can result in a penalty of up to $100 per day enforced by the Department of Labor.

Under ERISA, an employer is required to provide adequate notice to a plan participant whose claim for benefits has been denied. In the case of group health or disability plans, the notice must contain information about any internal rules, guidelines, or protocols that were relied upon when making the decision. The denial letter must outline "the specific reason for such denial, written in a manner calculated to be understood by the plan participant." For example, if the decision is based on a plan limitation that excludes treatments that are not medically necessary or are experimental, the notice must explain that scientific or clinical reason for the decision. In addition, the plan participant must be given "a reasonable opportunity for a full and fair review (ERISA Sec. 1133)."

Under ERISA regulations, a denial of any claim for benefits must be made "within a reasonable period of time." As a general rule, a period of more than 90 days is deemed unreasonable. If circumstances require a longer processing time, the plan may request an extension up to an additional 90 days after the participant has been given notice. When an urgent case is in need of an expedited decision, the plan must make its determination "as soon as possible, taking into account the medial exigencies" but no later than 72 hours after receipt of the claim unless the claim does not provide enough information to make a determination. The Department of Labor emphasizes that no time extensions are allowed in urgent cases. The determination of whether a claim is considered urgent can be made by a person acting on behalf of the plan "applying the judgment of a prudent layperson possessing an average knowledge of health and medicine." In addition, the plan must notify the patient within 45 days if a benefit claim is incomplete and specify the information required to complete the claim. The participant must be given at least 180 days to complete the claim. It is important that both the plan and the participant follow the deadlines given for appeal. In many cases, the plan will no longer view the case if the deadline has passed.

Contact ERISA

ERISA plans are enforced by the Department of Labor's Employee Benefits Security Administration (EBSA). You may contact your local office by calling 1-866-487-2365 or review plans at http://www.dol.gov/dol/topic/health-plans/erisa.htm. It is important to note that, under ERISA, if consumers are denied treatment, they may be able to collect punitive damages or compensation only if their state has mandated that right under state law.

Health Insurance Portability and Accountability Act (HIPAA)

HIPAA provides protections for beneficiaries covered by group health plans. It limits exclusions for pre-existing conditions. It prohibits discrimination against employees and dependents based on their health status, and it guarantees renewability and availability of health coverage to certain employees and individuals. To be protected under HIPAA, there cannot be a lapse or break in coverage of more than 63 days. Once members are no longer covered by a plan, they will be issued a certificate of credible coverage to provide to the new carrier. To learn more about your protections under HIPAA, visit http://www.dol.gov/dol/topic/health-plans/portability.htm .

Consolidated Omnibus Budget Reconciliation Act (COBRA)

Certain employers with 20 or more full-time employees or equivalent in the previous 12 months are required to offer continuation of coverage under COBRA to qualified beneficiaries. A qualified beneficiary is any individual, an employee, the employee's spouse, or an employee's dependent child, who was covered by the plan the day before the qualifying event. There are five qualifying events for which COBRA election would be necessary:

- Voluntary or involuntary termination of employment for reasons other than "gross misconduct"
- Reduction in the number of hours of employment
- Divorce or legal separation of the covered employee
- Death of the covered employee
- Loss of "dependent child" status under the plan rules.

Each beneficiary can elect COBRA independently. To learn more about your rights under COBRA, visit http://www.dol.gov/dol/topic/health-plans/cobra.htm .

Maintaining credible coverage is a concern for any individual, but if you have been diagnosed with a disease, it is crucial. Under HIPAA, beneficiaries covered by group health plans are safe-guarded. Under private or individual plans, the insurer may impose a complete pre-existing exclusion of anything related to your medical diagnosis. If you are facing coverage concerns, seek the assistance of a professional case manager at the Patient Advocate Foundation at 800-532-5274 or via the Internet at help@patientadvocate.org .

Medicaid

Medicaid is a federally funded, state-run program that provides medical assistance for individuals and families with limited income and resources that meet certain covered groups. Medicaid eligibility and coverage differs from state to state. There are many covered groups for Medicaid. Certain requirements must be met in order to be eligible for coverage, some of these include:

- Pregnant women
- Low-income families with children
- Aged, blind, and disabled
- SSI Eligible
- Emergency services for resident aliens/lawfully admitted immigrants
- Medically Needy Spend-Down Program

Check with your local social services agency to see whether you qualify for any of these programs. For many uninsured individuals, the cost of health insurance is prohibitive. Check with your local Medicaid office to find out whether your state offers a HIPP (Health Insurance Premium Payment) program.

Medicare beneficiaries of modest means may be eligible for one of the following Medicaid "Buy-In programs," these programs help pay all or some of Medicare's cost sharing amounts (i.e., premiums, deductibles, and copayments):

- **Qualified Medicare Beneficiary (QMB):** This program pays Medicare part A and/or B premiums, co-insurance and deductible for covered services for qualified individuals with incomes up to 100% of the Federal Poverty Guidelines (FPL).
- **Specified Low Income Medicare Beneficiary (SLMB):** This program pays Medicare part B premiums for qualified individuals with an income between 100% and 120% of the FPL and limited resources.
- **Qualified Individual program (QI):** This is an expansion of the SLMB program has that pays the Medicare part B monthly premium for qualified individuals with an income between 120% and 135% of the FPL. This program has a limited amount of funding, when funding is exhausted the benefit ends.
- **Qualified Disabled and Working Individual (QDWI):** States are required to pay the Medicare Part A premium for certain working disabled Medicare beneficiaries who have exhausted their entitlement to premium-free Part A benefits whose incomes does not exceed 200% of the FPL.

For more information, visit http://www.medicareadvocacy.org

If you lose your group health coverage benefits, check with your local Medicaid office to determine whether your children are eligible for coverage through SCHIPS (State Children's Health Insurance Program). This program is typically administered on a sliding fee scale, allowing parents to have a higher income. For more information, visit http://www.insurekidsnow.gov .

Financial Assistance

Individuals who do not have health insurance coverage and are in need of diagnostic services should contact their local health department. If you were diagnosed within a specific program, you may be entitled to immediate coverage through state or federal reimbursement programs.

If you have not yet started treatment, you may want to find a facility that offers charity care or has a financial assistance program. Call the billing office of a selected facility and ask whether they have a hardship, charity, or an indigent program. Programs are most likely offered through public hospitals and faith-based facilities. Be prepared to offer the facility details about your health and financial status.

There are programs available to assist you with getting your medications for free or at a reduced rate. Many medications are available through patient assistance programs offered by the pharmaceutical companies. Each company has its own eligibility requirements and application process. You can visit The Partnership for Prescription Assistance Web site, http://www.pparx .org/, for complete listings of drugs available through patient assistance programs.

The many facets of health care insurance discussed in this chapter are of great importance to the people of the United States, especially to the millions of patients and caregivers who are faced with illnesses and experience difficulty in accessing health care. In today's world, it is imperative that patients or caregivers be provided with information in order to make the right decisions that can ultimately affect the health, long-term insurability, and financial stability of the individual. The following resources are intended to help provide additional information on some of these facets of health care insurance.

Consumer Guides

The Georgetown University Health Policy Institute has written *A Consumer Guide to Getting and Keeping Health Insurance* for each state and Washington, DC. These guides summarize key consumer rights and protections in job-based group health insurance and individually purchased coverage. They also alert consumers to public programs in each state that may provide or subsidize health coverage. For more information, visit http:// www.healthinsuranceinfo.net .

Informative Web Sites:

Health care reform: http://www.insureUStoday.org

Usual, Customary & Reasonable Charges (UCR): http://www.patientadvocate.org/index.php?p=439

Government Web Sites

State insurance: http://www.naic.org/state_web_map.htm

ERISA: http://www.dol.gov/ebsa/compliance_assistance.html

COBRA: http://www.dol.gov/dol/topic/health-plans/cobra.htm

HIPAA: http://www.dol.gov/dol/topic/health-plans/portability.htm

Medicare and Medicaid: http://www.cms.hhs.gov

Health care reform: http://www.healthcare.gov

Cost-Sharing Assistance Charities

Assistance Fund
877-245-4412
http://theassistancefund.org

Cancer Care Co-Pay Assistance Fund
866-552-6729
http://www.cancercarecopay.org

Chronic Disease Fund
877-968-7233
http://www.cdfund.org

HealthWell Foundation
800-675-8416
http://www.healthwellfoundation.org

Leukemia & Lymphoma Society Co-Pay Assistance
877-557-2672
http://www.lls.org/copay

National Organization for Rare Disorders
866-828-8902
http://www.rarediseases.org

Patient Access Network
866-316-7263
https://www.panfoundation.org/

Patient Advocate Foundation Co-Pay Relief
866-512-3861
http://www.copays.org

Patient Services Inc.
800-366-7741
http://www.uneedpsi.org

Patient Assistance Programs:

RxAssist Patient Assistance Program Center
401-729-3284
http://www.rxassist.org

Partnership for Prescription Assistance
888-477-2669
http://www.pparx.org

NeedyMeds
http://www.needymeds.com

Together Rx Access
800-444-4106
http://www.togetherrxaccess.com

Selected References

Health Care Reform—The New York Times Web site. Retrieved August 01, 2010 from http://topics.nytimes.com/top/news/health/ diseasesconditionsandhealthtopics/health_insurance and_managed_care/health_care_reform/index.html.

Timeline: What's Changing and When. Retrieved July 31, 2010 from http://www.healthcare.gov/law/ timeline/index.html.

Timeline: When Health Care Reform Will Affect You. Retrieved June 23, 2010 from http://www.cnn. com/2010/POLITICS/03/23/health.care.timeline/ index.html.

5 Key Things to Remember about Health Care Reform: Retrieved April 30, 2010 from http:// www.cnn.com.

B. MEDICALLY NECESSARY DENTAL CARE

Mary Kaye Richter
Malinda Heuring

(Adapted from information prepared by the National
Foundation for Ectodermal Dysplasias)

"These charges are not covered under your medical plan. Please submit them to your dental carrier." How familiar these words are to the oral and head and neck cancer survivor who is undergoing rehabilitative treatment by an oral surgeon, dentist, or prosthodontist to restore functions of speech and mastication to an acceptable state.

The fact that the patient was diagnosed with oral and head and neck cancer and that the dental problems and rehabilitation program occurred as a result of necessary medical treatment for the cancer is often lost as insurance companies attempt to fit the patient into the "mold" that has been created. Granted, under normal circumstances dental services and supplies provided by the dental team are excluded from medical insurance plans; however, in cases in which dental care is necessitated by a treatment and/or surgery for a medical problem, there should be no question of medical insurance benefits.

Oral and head and neck cancer patients have a wide range of challenges they must address during their cancer journey. One of these challenges is dental care and proving that the care is medically necessary and therefore covered under a medical insurance policy. Proving that dental care is medically necessary is not easy. It is helpful to have a record of having received medical benefits for oral and head and neck cancer treatments prior to seeking dental benefits under the medical policy. Begin your quest with the very first visit to the dentist.

When dealing with your insurer, it is important to keep detailed records. Start a notebook that will allow you to document all telephone conservations with the insurance company. Request that all rulings be made in writing and file this documentation with your notebook. The process ahead may not be an easy one, but keeping duplicates of all letters and notes from all telephone conversations with the insurance company could ultimately prove helpful.

The first request for dental benefits from a medical insurance carrier is almost always denied. Typically, these requests are received by a clerk who is familiar with the policy language.

Because dental benefits are routinely excluded, the clerk will indicate that benefits do not apply and a denial will follow. You need this denial in writing. Under the Employee Retirement and Income Security Act (ERISA), your denial letter should include a for the denial and a reference to your plan explaining the basis for the denial. After you receive this documentation, you can start the appeals process. When you appeal, you should immediately ask that a case manager handle your requests. A case manager is more capable of handling complex benefit questions.

Sometimes the process must be repeated . . . and repeated . . . and repeated. The average insurance clerk is not familiar with oral and head and neck cancer and serves the company not the consumer. It is important that the company understand that you will not give up until an appropriate decision is made. This can take many, many months. Customers are likely to either accept the initial denial or get tired of the fight. If success seems out of reach, the assistance of an attorney may be helpful. It doesn't take an insurer long to figure out that legal bills will quickly exceed the cost of a set of dentures and that it may be easier to pay the latter rather than the former. In addition, the situation could turn into a public relations nightmare for the company.

In either event, it is of the utmost importance that the insurance company be made to understand that oral and head and neck cancer and its treatments of radiation therapy and chemotherapy may result in dental problems and therefore the dental treatment for those problems should be considered a component of care necessitated by a medical condition.

If you receive insurance through an employer, be familiar with the type of insurance you have. Call the human resources manager or office manager and ask for that person's help in explaining your coverage. If the employer is self-insured, the employer typically hires a third party to administer the plan and the company pays the claims. This has its advantages and disadvantages.

If your company is self-insured, your company does not have to comply with the health insurance regulations in your state pursuant to ERISA. The employer can choose to pay a claim that typically is not a covered benefit. Work with the human resources department and explain your situation, both verbally and in writing. The company may choose to pay the claim, or the human resources department may be able to put pressure on the insurance carrier to get the claim approved.

After your initial request results in a denial, you should appeal this decision. The denial letter will include the steps you need to take if you disagree with the decision. Typically you have two written appeals and one in-person or over-the-phone appeal. For the first appeal, put together a packet of information for the insurance company that includes supporting documentation to combat the insurance company's reason for denial. This documentation should include letters from all care providers (physicians, dentists, and so on) who are directly involved with your care, indicating that the oral treatment needs are a direct result of the treatment for cancer.

At this point make sure the policy language in your policy booklet is consistent with the insurance company's reason for denial. Insurance companies have been known to deny benefits even though the benefits should be covered as stated in the policy booklet.

Be sure to keep copies of everything you send to your insurance company. Mail the appeal certified mail. Insurance companies "lose" documentation quite often. If your first appeal is not successful, you can submit much of the same information with your second appeal.

Documents should include the following:

■ An appeal letter telling the insurance company why you disagree with its decision and why it should cover your needed dental work. Include factual information and any documented research. Be sure to include all of your identification numbers (policy number, group number, claim number, and so on) in this letter. Request that the denial be reviewed by the insurance company's medical review board (MRB). All insurance companies have MRBs because the expertise of physicians/dentists is needed in special circumstances. The letter should also include a short history of your struggles with oral and head and neck cancer. Finally, include a statement asking the insurance company to overturn its denial and approve your claim.

■ A letter from your dentist and oral specialist addressing specifics of your case.

■ A letter from your medical physician stating that dental issues can be the result of treatment for oral and head and neck cancer.

■ Any important information from your medical records along with copies of similar claims the medical insurance has previously paid.

The next step is to wait for a response from the insurance company. If you get a positive response, celebrate! Make sure that you get this response in writing and that you are aware of any conditions attached to this approval. If the response is negative, appeal to the next level.

Never fail to be optimistic; you must convince the insurance carrier that there is *no doubt* that you *will win* and you will *not stop* until you reach a satisfactory resolution. Make your presence known. Make it a priority to speak to those capable of resolving the issue, or at the very least, have direct access to those with the power to make it happen. Be organized and be prepared! Always let the insurance company know that you may understand their position; however, you *do not agree* with it.

Let them know you are listening but that you expect them to reciprocate and actually what you are saying. Be pleasant, but . Remind them of their own children and grandchildren; believe it or not, they are people just like us. Be committed because this will take time and endless energy. Believe in yourself and know the result will be worth the many hours of effort, frustration, anger, resentment, and anxiety you have experienced.

Useful Tips

- Follow up all telephone calls with a letter stating what was talked about so that you have a written record.
- Don't send more information than is asked for.
- Look for flaws in the denial language.
- Get the insurance company mission statement and use it against the company.
- Challenge everything.
- Appeal to the highest level.
- Request a specialist.
- Inform the insurance company of other medical problems related to oral and head and neck cancer that it has paid for (dermatologist, ENT, and so on).
- Don't give up.
- File your claim on a medical claim form, not a dental claim form.
- Find out the medical diagnosis codes for your particular claim.

C. EVERYTHING YOU NEED TO KNOW ABOUT OBTAINING SOCIAL SECURITY DISABILITY BENEFITS

Scott E. Davis, Disability Attorney

If you have paid taxes to the federal government, part of these taxes purchased a disability policy from the Social Security Administration (SSA). Everyone understands they are entitled to *retirement* benefits from SSA, but many people do not understand they also have *disability* insurance through SSA. Many people mistakenly believe by seeking disability benefits they are "living off the government" if they file a disability claim and receive benefits. It is important to move quickly past this erroneous belief because SSA sold all of us a disability policy and "you better use it" or you may lose it.

Receiving disability benefits from SSA plays an important role in your recovery because it eases the considerable stress that results when and if you are unable to work because of your medical condition.

Not Filing a Claim Brings Devastating Financial Consequences

Unfortunately, not filing a disability claim with SSA when you should brings devastating financial consequences. Many reasons exist to file, foremost that filing a claim protects your earnings record for retirement. Your SSA retirement benefit is based on annual earnings; if you are disabled and not paying social security taxes, then "zeroes" are posted each year to your SSA earnings record. If you are disabled but *do not* file a disability claim, SSA does not know you are disabled and assumes you decided to stop working. SSA then includes the nonearning disability years to your overall earnings record, which potentially reduces your retirement benefit significantly because your SSA earnings record was not protected during the time you were disabled.

A major benefit of being found disabled by SSA is that it protects your earnings record. Beginning with the year you are found disabled, SSA protects your record by not adding in any of the nonearning years when calculating your retirement benefit. The result is if you remain disabled through retirement age, there is no reduction between your disability and retirement benefit. You must apply for Social Security Disability Insurance (SSDI) before you file for early retirement. You will get whichever benefit is higher, not both.

How Does SSA Define Disability?

SSA's definition of disability is easier to meet than most people realize. Many people mistakenly believe you need a catastrophic injury or need to be confined to a wheelchair or be "permanently" disabled to be eligible. These misconceptions are the reasons that many people do not file a claim, erroneously believing their medical condition is not severe enough to qualify for benefits. Simply put, you qualify for disability benefits if, as a result of any physical or psychological medical condition (or both), you are unable to work in any occupation for a minimum of 12 consecutive months, or your condition is expected to result in death.

As long as you or your doctors expect that you will be unable to work in any occupation for *at least 12 months*, then you are eligible for benefits. Permanent disability is not required. Many cancer patients are or can be disabled for several years, receive benefits while recovering from residual effects of treatment, and then eventually return to work.

When to File a Claim

File your claim as soon as you or your doctors believe you meet SSA's definition of disability. If your diagnosis is not treatable and is expected to result in death, immediately file your claim and send the information supporting the diagnosis (i.e., pathology reports, lab results, medical records with clinical findings, and so on) to SSA. Be sure to tell SSA personnel of your condition and ask them to declare your case a "TERI" case. TERI stands for "terminal illness." A TERI case receives expedited claim processing. However, it will be up to you to bring the severity of your condition to SSA's attention; don't assume SSA will do anything.

If your condition is treatable, you might want to continue working as long as you can while receiving treatment because many people find it therapeutic. However, if side effects or residual effects of treatment begin to significantly affect your ability to work on a consistent, daily basis or have an adverse impact on your prognosis, you should file your claim once you have stopped working or expect to be unable to work for a minimum of 12 consecutive months.

At the Latest, File Your Disability Claim Within 5 Years of Being Disabled

You become insured for SSA disability benefits by paying social security taxes for at least 5 of the 10 years *before becoming disabled*. It is critical to understand that SSA's disability insurance does not last forever—you must use it or you eventually lose it. To avoid losing your insurance, be sure to file your claim within 5 years of becoming disabled. File your claim by calling Social Security at 800-772-1213, visiting a local office, or going online at http://www.ssa.gov . There is no charge to file a claim.

Benefits You Will Receive

In addition to protecting your earnings record for retirement, you will receive a monthly monetary payment that varies based on your SSA earnings record. You will also receive Medicare health insurance 29 months after you are first eligible for benefits.

Appeal If Your Claim Is Denied

It is *critical* to appeal if SSA denies your claim. Many people mistakenly believe SSA represents them and will assist in the approval of their claim. The truth is SSA initially denies significantly more claims than it approves. With regard to cancer claims, SSA frequently views *any* initial positive responses to treatment to mean the person can work or return to work. SSA also routinely ignores the residual effects of treatment, preferring instead to focus on response and stage of disease.

Incredibly, SSA statistics confirm that 50% of the time people never appeal the initial denial of their claim. Please avoid becoming a statistic by appealing every denial within 60 days of the date stamped on the denial. It is also critical to not lose hope because eventually the overwhelming majority of claims are approved.

How Social Security Evaluates Head and Neck Cancer

There are several ways SSA can approve a disability claim based on head and neck cancer.

1. **Based on severity of the disease.** Your claim can be approved based solely on the diagnosis depending on the stage of disease. Head and neck cancer falls under Social Security's "Listed Impairments," meaning the law requires your claim to be approved if the stage of disease meets the listed criteria. The specific Adult Listing 13.02 for soft tissue tumors of the head and neck (except salivary glands and thyroid gland, which are listed separately elsewhere) includes the following disease criteria ("Disability Evaluation," 2006):

   A. Inoperable or unresectable.

   B. Persistent disease following initial multimodal antineoplastic therapy.

   C. Recurrent disease following initial antineoplastic therapy, except local vocal cord recurrence.

   D. With metastases beyond the regional lymph nodes.

   E. Soft tissue tumors of the head and neck not addressed in A–D, with multimodal antineoplastic therapy. Consider under a disability until at least 18 months from the date of diagnosis. Thereafter, evaluate any residual impairment(s) under the criteria for the affected body system. If the stage of your disease meets any of these criteria, SSA *must* approve your claim.

2. **Based on inability to sustain work.** What if your condition does not meet SSA's listed criteria? If your diagnosis does not meet the criteria, you can still be approved for disability benefits. Most cancer diagnoses initially will not meet SSA's listed criteria because the listed criteria represent an advanced stage of disease. You are eligible for benefits if you have significant residual effects from cancer treatment or have other medical conditions in addition to the cancer that contribute to your inability to work.

As a general rule, if you do not meet SSA's listed criteria, you must be unable to sustain *sedentary* work on a regular and continuous basis (i.e., SSA defines this as 8 hours per day, 5 days per week) to be eligible. Claims that are based on cancer are often approved because individuals are unable to sustain work due to the cumulative effects of treatment even though the stage of their disease is not advanced enough to meet SSA's listed criteria.

For example, after undergoing radiation and/or chemotherapy, a person's physical and mental stamina can be significantly diminished. Also, the *desire* to communicate and the ability to effectively deal with any stress can be significantly reduced, making consistent work impossible. Furthermore, taking high-dose narcotics for pain control can cause exhaustion and cognitive dysfunction, which further erode stamina and the ability to attend and concentrate.

Because the cumulative effects of cancer treatment can pose significant work limitations, the prudent course is to file your disability claim *sooner rather than later*. When should you file your disability claim? You should do so either when: (a) you meet SSA's listed criteria as set forth previously, or (b) you do not meet the criteria but you or your doctors believe you will be unable to sustain full-time work for a minimum of 12 months. Remember, if you are able to return to work after treatment, you can always tell SSA you seek benefits only for the period of time you were off work as long as it lasted more than 12 months, or withdraw your claim altogether if you return to work within 12 months of your initial disability.

Remember to Consider Other Diagnoses That May Preclude Work

Following a cancer diagnosis or after beginning treatment, depression and anxiety may pose significant problems in returning to work. Depression and anxiety, alone or in combination with other limitations resulting from cancer, can be disabling. An example would be a person who has developed significant secondary psychological problems even though that person's cancer treatment appears to have been successful.

Also, if you have undergone invasive oral surgery and are unable to consistently use your voice (or cannot communicate easily), need special accommodations (i.e., a feeding tube), or must take strong narcotics for pain control, you should be eligible for disability benefits.

Hire an Attorney Who Specializes in Social Security Law

SSA's own statistics (Attorney Fee Payment, 2001) prove that one way to significantly increase the odds of obtaining disability benefits is by hiring an experienced social security disability attorney. Consult with and hire an attorney as soon as you believe you may not be able to continue working. Social security attorneys work on a contingency fee, meaning you pay a fee only if your claim is approved and you receive monetary benefits. The attorney should be experienced in social security law because the area is complex and it is easy to make costly mistakes.

Attorney's fees in social security cases are regulated by federal law and almost every attorney uses a standard contingency fee agreement in which the fee is 25% of all past due monetary benefits or $6,000, whichever is the lesser amount. For example, if you have $10,000 in past due benefits when the claim is approved, the fee is $2,500; if you have $40,000 in past due benefits, the maximum fee you pay is $6,000.

An attorney will work directly with SSA personnel so you do not have to. This allows you to focus on recovery. An attorney should also help you complete SSA's forms and will develop medical evidence from your physicians regarding whether you meet SSA's listed criteria. An attorney knows the specific work limitations that are important to obtain from your physician to help prove you are unable to work. SSA generally does not obtain this critical evidence; it simply processes your case and evaluates your ability to work based solely on your medical records.

The following list includes resources for additional information if you are considering applying for disability insurance.

- http://www.scottdavispc.com: Web site of the author where you can find many practical articles concerning disability benefits
- http://www.ssa.gov: Web site of the Social Security Administration
- http://www.nosscr.org: Web site of the National Organization of Social Security Claimants' Representatives from which you can obtain a referral to an experienced social security disability attorney
- http://www.severe.net: Web site of Social Security Disability Benefits Law Information and Resources (Severe.net), hosted by experienced social security attorneys with a wealth of disability information and links to resources.

In summary, all people who have paid taxes to the federal government are eligible for retirement benefits and disability insurance. The information provided here is intended to serve as a guide to help you avoid mistakes in seeking disability benefits and help you find the information you need. It is of utmost importance that you not become discouraged during the process of seeking disability benefits and that you follow through with persistence, keeping your spirits high while fighting for the benefits for which you are entitled.

References

Attorney Fee Payment System Improvement Act 2001. *Congressional Record,* November 16, 2001 (testimony of Honorable Robert T. Matsui and Honorable E. Clay Shaw).

Disability evaluation under social security. (2006, June). *Blue book.* Available at http://www.ssa.gov/disability/professionals/bluebook .

15

MEETING THE CHALLENGES OF CLINICAL TRIALS

A. CLINICAL TRIALS

Nancy E. Leupold, MA

(Adapted from the National Cancer Institute's
Educational Materials About Clinical Trials)

Clinical trials, also called research studies, test new treatments in people with cancer. The goal of this research is to find better methods to treat cancer and help cancer patients. Clinical trials seek to answer specific scientific questions to find better ways to prevent, detect, and treat diseases and to improve care for people with diseases. Clinical trials may test many types of treatment such as new drugs, new approaches to surgery or radiation therapy, new combinations of treatments, or new methods such as gene therapy. A clinical trial is one of the final stages of a long and careful research process. The search for new treatments begins in the laboratory, where scientists first develop and test new ideas. If an approach seems promising, the next step may be testing a treatment in animals to see how it affects cancer in a living being and whether it has harmful effects. Of course, treatments that work well in the lab or in animals do not always work well in people. Studies are done with cancer patients to find out whether promising treatments are safe and effective.

Types of Clinical Trials

There are several different types of cancer clinical trials. Each type of trial is designed to answer different research questions.

- **Prevention trials** test new approaches, such as medicines, vitamins, minerals, or other supplements that doctors believe may lower the risk of a certain type of cancer. These trials are designed to find the best way to prevent cancer in people who have never had cancer or to prevent cancer from coming back or a new cancer occurring in people who have already had cancer.
- **Screening trials** are designed to find the best way to detect cancer in its early stages, before symptoms develop. These trials involve people who do not have any symptoms of cancer.
- **Diagnostic trials** study tests or procedures that could be used to identify cancer more accurately. Diagnostic trials usually include people who have signs or symptoms of cancer.
- **Treatment trials** are conducted with people who have cancer. They test new treatments such as a new cancer drug, new approaches to surgery or radiation therapy, new combinations

of treatments, or new methods such as gene therapy. These trials are designed to find out what new treatment approaches can help people who have cancer and what the most effective treatment is for people who have cancer.

■ **Quality of life trials** (also called supportive care trials) are designed to explore ways to improve comfort and quality of life for people who have cancer. These trials may study ways to help people who are experiencing side effects from cancer or its treatment.

■ **Genetics studies** are sometimes part of another cancer clinical trial. The genetics component of the trial may focus on how genetic makeup can affect detection, diagnosis, or response to cancer treatment. Population- and family-based genetic research studies differ from traditional cancer clinical trials. In these studies, researchers look at tissue or blood samples, generally from families or large groups of people, to find genetic changes that are associated with cancer. People who participate in genetics studies may or may not have cancer, depending on the study. The goal of these studies is to help understand the role of genes in the development of cancer.

How Patients Are Protected

Clinical trials are conducted in doctors' offices, cancer centers, other medical centers, community hospitals and clinics, and veterans' and military hospitals in cities and towns across the United States and in other countries. Clinical trials may include participants at one or two highly specialized centers, or they may involve hundreds of locations at the same time.

Doctors, nurses, social workers, and other health professionals are part of the treatment team. They will monitor the patient's progress closely. Patients may have more tests and doctor visits than if they were not taking part in a study. Each patient will follow a treatment plan prescribed by the doctor. Patients may also have other responsibilities such as keeping a log or filling out forms about their health. Some studies continue to check on patients even after their treatment is over.

In clinical trials, both research concerns and patient well-being are important. To help protect patients and produce sound results, research with people is carried out according to strict scientific and ethical principles, which include the following:

- **Each clinical trial has an action plan (protocol) that explains how it will work.** The study's investigator, usually a doctor, prepares an action plan for the study. Known as a protocol, this plan explains what will be done in the study and why. It outlines how many people will take part in the study, what medical tests they will receive and how often, and the treatment plan. Each doctor who takes part uses the same protocol. For patient safety, each protocol must be approved by the organization that sponsors the study (such as the National Cancer Institute) and the Institutional Review Board (IRB) at each hospital or other study site. This board, which includes consumers, clergy, and health professionals, reviews the protocol to be sure that the research will not expose patients to extreme or unethical risks.

- **Each study enrolls people who are alike in key ways.** Each study's protocol describes the characteristics that all patients in the study must have. Called eligibility criteria, these guidelines differ from study to study, depending on the research purpose. They may include age, gender, the type and stage of cancer, and whether cancer patients who have had prior cancer treatment or who have other health problems can take part.

  Using eligibility criteria is an important principle of medical research that helps produce reliable results. During a study, they help protect patient safety so that people who are likely to be harmed by study drugs or other treatments are not exposed to the risk. After results are in, they also help doctors know which patient groups will benefit if the new treatment being studied is proved to work. For instance, a new treatment may work for one type of cancer but not another, or it may be more effective for men than women.

- **The informed consent process is an integral part of research.** Informed consent, a legal, regulatory, and ethical concept, is the process of learning the key facts about a clinical trial before deciding whether to participate. It is also a continuing process throughout the study to provide information for participants. To help someone decide whether or not to participate, the doctors and nurses involved in the trial explain the details of the study. If the participant's native language is not English, translation assistance can be provided. Then the research team provides an informed consent document that includes details about the study, such as its purpose, duration, required procedures, and key contacts. Risks and potential benefits are explained in this document. The participant then decides whether or not to sign the document. The process does not end with the signing of informed consent documents. If new benefits, risks, or side effects are discovered during the trial, researchers must inform participants. Informed consent is not a contract, and the participant may withdraw from the trial at any time. Participants are encouraged to ask questions at any time.

Cancer clinical trials are usually conducted in a series of steps, called *phases*. Treatment clinical trials are always assigned a phase. However, screening, prevention, diagnostic, and quality-of-life studies do not always have a phase nor do genetics clinical trials.

Each phase answers different questions about the new treatment.

- *Phase I* trials are the first step in testing a new treatment in humans. In these studies, researchers look for the best way to give a new treatment (e.g., by mouth, IV drip, or injection and number of times a day). They also try to find out if and how the treatment can be given safely (e.g., best dose), and they watch for any harmful side effects. Because less is known about the possible risks and benefits in phase I, these studies usually include only a limited number of patients, between 15 and 30, who would not be helped by other known treatments.
- *Phase II* trials continue to test the safety of the new agent and begin to evaluate how well it works against a specific type of cancer. As in phase I, only a small number of people (fewer than 100) take part. In general, these participants have been treated with chemotherapy, surgery, or radiation, but treatment has not been effective. It is important to remember that, when a phase II trial begins, it is not yet known if the agent tested works against the specific cancer being studied. Unpredictable side effects can also occur in these trials.

■ *Phase III* trials focus on how a new treatment compares with standard treatment (treatment currently accepted and most widely used). Researchers want to learn whether the new treatment is better than, the same as, or worse than the standard treatment. They assign patients by chance either to a group taking the new treatment (called the treatment group) or to a group taking standard treatment (called the control group). This method, called randomization, helps avoid bias (having the study's results affected by human choices or other factors not related to the treatments being tested).

Comparing similar groups of people taking different treatments for the same type of cancer is another way to make sure that study results are real and caused by the treatment rather than by chance or other factors. Comparing treatments with each other often shows clearly which one is more effective or has fewer side effects.

In most cases, studies move into phase III testing only after a treatment shows promise in phases I and II. Phase III trials may include hundreds to thousands of people around the country (and world) ranging from people newly diagnosed with cancer to people with extensive disease.

■ *Phase IV* trials are used to further evaluate the long-term safety and effectiveness of a treatment. Less common than phase I, II, and III trials, phase IV trials usually take place after the new treatment has been approved for standard use.

Benefits and Risks of Participating in a Clinical Trial

Although a clinical trial is a good choice for some people, this treatment option has possible benefits and drawbacks.

Possible Benefits

■ Clinical trials offer high-quality (high-quality is somewhat subjective) cancer care.

■ Participants receive regular and careful medical attention from a research team that includes doctors and other health professionals.

■ Participants have access to promising new approaches that are often not available outside the clinical trial setting.

■ The approach being studied may be more effective than the standard approach.

■ Participants may be the first to benefit from the new method under study.

■ Results from the study may help others in the future.

Possible Drawbacks

■ New drugs or procedures under study are not always better than, or even as good as, standard care.

■ New treatments may have side effects that doctors do not expect or that are worse than those of standard treatment

■ Participants in randomized trials will not be able to choose the approach they receive.

■ Even standard treatments, proved effective for many people, do not help everyone.

■ Health insurance and managed care providers do not always cover all patient care costs in a study.

■ The protocol may require more time and attention than would a nonprotocol treatment, including trips to the study site, more treatments, hospital stays, or complex dosage requirements.

To find answers to questions about how clinical trials work and patients' rights and protections, consult a doctor, nurse, or other health care professional.

Where to Find Information About Clinical Trials

■ **NCI-sponsored clinical trial programs:** http://www.cancer.gov/clinicaltrials

■ **National Institute of Health (NIH) clinical trials:** http://www.clinicaltrials.gov

■ **National Cancer Institute Clinical Trials Education Series:** http://www.cancer.gov/clinicaltrials/education/clinical-trials-education-series

■ **National Library of Medicine:** http://www.nlm.nih.gov/ offers links to resources for finding the results of clinical trials. It includes information about published and unpublished results. http://www.nlm.nih.gov/services/ctresults.html

■ **TrialCheck:** http://www.trialcheck.org/Services/ is a search tool developed and maintained by the Coalition of Cancer Cooperative Groups. It consists of groups of doctors and other health professionals that carry out many of the larger cancer clinical trials in the United States that are funded by the National Cancer Institute. This search tool uses nine simple questions. After patients answer these questions, they will receive a list of cancer clinical trials in which they may be eligible to enroll. TrialCheck also allows a patient to search for a cancer clinical trial at specific locations.

■ **EmergingMed:** http://www.emergingmed.com/ is a free and confidential cancer clinical trial matching and referral service. Patients and caregivers can find matches to clinical trials by calling toll free to speak with patient support specialists (877-601-8601) or by visiting the Emerging-Med Web site. Patients will be encouraged to identify their clinical trial options and then review them with their doctor whenever a treatment decision is necessary. EmergingMed's patient support specialists are available Monday through Friday, 8:30 AM to 6 PM EST.

Costs Associated with a Clinical Trial

Health insurance and managed care providers often do not cover the patient care costs associated with a clinical trial. What they cover varies by health plan and by study. Some health plans do not cover clinical trials if they consider the approach being studied "experimental" or "investigational." However, if enough data show that the approach is safe and effective, a health plan may consider the approach "established" and cover some or all of the costs.

Participants may have difficulty obtaining coverage for costs associated with prevention and screening clinical trials; health plans are currently less likely to have review processes in place for these studies. Therefore, it may be more difficult to get coverage for the costs associated with them. In many cases, it helps to have someone from the research team talk about coverage with representatives of the health plan.

Health plans may specify other criteria that a trial must meet to be covered. The trial might have to be sponsored by a specified organization, be judged "medically necessary" by the health plan, not be significantly more expensive than treatments the health plan considers standard, or focus on types of cancer for which no standard treatments are available. In addition, the facility and medical staff might have to meet the plan's qualifications for conducting certain procedures, such as bone marrow transplants. More information about insurance coverage can be found on the NCI's *Clinical Trials and Insurance Coverage: A Resource Guide* Web page at http://www.cancer.gov/clinical trials/learning/insurance-coverage .

Many states have passed legislation or developed policies requiring health plans to cover the costs of certain clinical trials. For more information, visit the NCI's Web site at http://www.cancer .gov/clinicaltrials/developments/laws-about-clinical-trial-costs.

Federal programs that help pay the costs of care in a clinical trial include the following:

■ Medicare reimburses patient care costs for its beneficiaries who participate in clinical trials designed to diagnose or treat cancer. Information about Medicare coverage of clinical trials is available at http://www.medicare.gov, or by calling Medicare's toll-free number for beneficiaries at 800-633-4227 (800-MEDI-CARE). The toll-free number for the hearing impaired is 877-486-2048. Also, the NCI fact sheet, *More Choices in Cancer Care: Information for Beneficiaries on Medicare Coverage of*

Cancer Clinical Trials is available at http://www.cancer.gov/cancertopics/factsheet/support/medicare .

■ Beneficiaries of TRICARE, the Department of Defense's health program, can be reimbursed for the medical costs of participation in NCI-sponsored phase II and phase III cancer prevention (including screening and early detection) and treatment trials. Additional information is available in the NCI fact sheet, *TRICARE Beneficiaries Can Enter Clinical Trials for Cancer Prevention and Treatment Through a Department of Defense and National Cancer Institute Agreement.* This fact sheet can be found at http://www.cancer.gov/cancertopics/factsheet/NCI/TRICARE .

■ The Department of Veterans Affairs (VA) allows eligible veterans to participate in NCI-sponsored prevention, diagnosis, and treatment studies nationwide. All phases and types of NCI-sponsored trials are included. The NCI fact sheet, *The NCI/VA Agreement on Clinical Trials: Questions and Answers,* has more information. It is available at http://www.cancer.gov/cancertopics/factsheet/NCI/VA-clinical-trials.

Completion of a Clinical Trial

After a clinical trial is completed, the researchers look carefully at the data collected during the trial before making decisions about the meaning of the findings and further testing. After a phase I or II trial, the researchers decide whether to move on to the next phase, or stop testing the agent or intervention because it was not safe or effective. When a phase III trial is completed, the researchers look at the data and decide whether the results have medical importance.

The results of clinical trials are often published in peer-reviewed, scientific journals. Peer review is a process by which experts review the report before it is published to make sure the analysis and conclusions are sound. If the results are particularly important, they may be featured by the media and discussed at scientific meetings and by patient advocacy groups before they are published. Once a new approach has proved safe and effective in a clinical trial, it may become standard practice (standard practice is a currently accepted and widely used approach).

B. FINDING A CLINICAL TRIAL TO MEET YOUR SPECIFIC NEEDS

Patty Delaney
Deborah J. Miller, PhD, MPH, RN

Finding a clinical trial to meet the specific needs of a patient can be a challenge. Unfortunately, there are many formidable barriers that impede patient access to cancer clinical trials. Physicians may be resistant to referring patients to clinical trials, and health insurance may not always cover expenses incurred during participation in a clinical trial. There may be restrictions on eligibility that prohibit participation in a clinical trial, or an individual who is interested in participating in a study may be concerned about receiving a placebo and not the drug being tested. In addition, individuals may have fears about being randomized to receive a treatment that is perceived to be less aggressive than the new unproven treatment. Last, individuals may have difficulty locating a clinical trial that meets their needs and may find a daunting challenge in contacting clinical trial sites to learn about the clinical trial status and their eligibility.

The Internet has made a huge difference in improving access to information on cancer clinical trials. The Internet provides sources of information about cancer clinical trials being conducted by a variety of institutions and individuals, including hospitals, drug companies, private doctors, and the government.

The passage of the Food and Drug Administration Modernization Act of 1997 directed the Secretary of Health and Human Services, acting through the Director of National Institutes of Health (NIH), to establish, maintain, and operate a data bank of information on clinical trials for drugs to treat serious or life-threatening diseases and conditions. This database was intended to be a central resource, providing current information on clinical trials to individuals, other members of the public, and health care providers and researchers.

NIH, through its National Library of Medicine and with input from the Food and Drug Administration (FDA) and others, developed the Clinical Trials Data Bank at http://www.clinical trials.gov. The first version of this data bank was made available to the public on February 29, 2000. At that time, the data bank included primarily NIH-sponsored clinical trials. In March of the same year, FDA issued guidelines to members of the pharmaceutical industry that outlined when and how they were to list their clinical trials on the site. When the sponsor of a clinical trial begins to investigate whether its drug is effective (phase II, III, and IV clinical trials) in serious and life-threatening diseases and conditions, the clinical trial's sponsor, including drug companies, academic medical centers, or individual doctors, must list that phase II, III, or IV trial in http://www.clinicaltrials.gov . The clinical trial sponsors must list the following information:

- Purpose of the clinical trial
- Patient eligibility criteria
- Location of the clinical trial sites
- Telephone number and name of a contact person.

Prior to 2007, not all cancer clinical trials being conducted by pharmaceutical companies and academic medical centers were listed in clinicaltrials.gov, but the passage of the Food and Drug Administration Amendments Act of 2007 required *all* clinical trials studying the effectiveness of a drug to be listed on http://www.clinicaltrials.gov. Additionally, this act expanded the data bank to include results of clinical trials.

Other sources for clinical trials include newspaper articles, medical journals, not-for-profit and for-profit Web sites, as well as the Web sites of individual pharmaceutical companies.

With so much information available, how does one find the latest drugs being studied specifically for oral and head and neck cancer?

Following are some sources of information that may be helpful in finding a clinical trial to fit a patient's needs.

- **National Institutes of Health (NIH) Web site: http://www. clinicaltrials.gov.** The fact that this clinical trials Web site exists at all is due exclusively to the patient advocacy community, especially cancer patient advocates. The patient advocates lobbied Congress to make it a requirement that drug companies add their clinical trials of drugs for serious and life-threatening diseases and conditions to a publicly accessible database as soon as the drug companies begin to investigate the effectiveness of their unapproved drug. Investigations of a drug's effectiveness usually begin at phase II, after the phase I to define the pharmacokinetics (absorption, distribution, metabolism, and excretion) of a drug in the body, and decide on appropriate dosing clinical trials have been completed. The site affords search options that permit patients to find clinical trials for specific diseases and conditions, such as head and neck cancers, as well as specific geographical areas.

■ **National Cancer Institute's (NCI) Web site: http://www .cancer.gov/clinicaltrials**. The NCI clinical trial database can be searched by selecting a specific cancer from a list on its Website. NCI also maintains a valuable clinical trial telephone service. It also can be accessed by telephone at 800-4-CANCER.

■ **American Cancer Society's (ACS) Web site: http://www .cancer.org**. This site provides a confidential matching service for clinical trials nationwide as well as other clinical trial information. To access the Web page, search for "clinical trials."

■ **Support for People with Oral and Head and Neck Cancer (SPOHNC) Web site: http://www.spohnc.org**. This site provides access to clinical trials information. Select "Clinical Trials" under Cancer Information on the home page. The clinical trials listed on this Web site are those related to oral and head and neck cancer. On this Web page, you will find different types of clinical trials, what happens in them, the clinical trial process, information on clinical trial phases, and more.

■ **Pharmaceutical Research and Manufacturers of America (PhRMA) Web site: http://www.phrma.org**. This site has clinical trials information listed under the tab Research. This Web site is the drug industry's trade association. It lists new drugs that are in development and the name of the company developing the drug.

■ **Coalition of Cancer Cooperative Groups (CCCG) Web site: http://www.cancertrialshelp.org**. The Coalition of Cancer Cooperative Groups is the nation's premier network of cancer clinical trials specialists. Its diverse, comprehensive membership includes all 10 of the nation's federally funded cancer Cooperative Groups (large networks of researchers, physicians, and healthcare professionals across the country who are working to improve the quality of life and survival of cancer patients by increasing participation in cancer clinical trials), the country's leading patient advocacy organizations, and oncology and cancer research specialists.

Although the Internet is a valuable resource, it often is not interactive. For example, if the information in the clinical trial listing is unclear, it may not be possible to have your specific questions answered online and in a timely manner. However, a telephone number is usually included in the clinical trial listing, and you may be able to get answers to specific questions about a given clinical trial by calling the number listed.

Researching a Clinical Trial That Is Right for You

Before deciding on a specific clinical trial to meet your needs, you should take the following steps to understand your diagnosis, treatment options, and the clinical trials that may be available to you.

Step 1. Learn as much about your disease and diagnosis as you possibly can—for example, the specific type of cancer, the stage of the disease, the size of the tumor, the cell type, the tumor locations, and the standard treatment for your diagnosis. If the diagnosis is a recurrence, you should have a record available of your previous treatment, including the drug names, dates of treatment and the number of treatments, and the location and extent of the recurrence.

Step 2. Write down your diagnosis and treatment information or type it into a computer and keep it accessible in a file you can easily consult. Remember to always have this information with you when you are inquiring about a clinical trial. Practice reporting a summary of your diagnosis with a relative or friend. You should be able to recount your diagnosis in a few minutes, similar to the way one doctor might report your diagnosis to another doctor, with no extraneous information, just the facts. For example: "I was 50 years old when I was diagnosed with stage III squamous cell carcinoma of the base of the tongue.

I had 36 external beam radiation therapy treatments coupled with weekly chemotherapy. The tumor on my tongue shrunk and what remained was surgically removed along with some malignant lymph nodes. It is now a year and a half since my surgery, and I have just been diagnosed with a recurrence of the cancer. I am now looking for a clinical trial."

Step 3. Ask your doctor's staff for assistance if you are uncertain about the details of your diagnosis. Remember that information in your medical record can easily be obtained by the staff in your doctor's office. You do not have to take your doctor's time to make this request.

Step 4. Let your doctor know you are investigating clinical trial options. Physicians, especially oncologists, are extremely busy and may not have the time or staff available to explore this option with you. However, your doctor should know that you are pursuing this option and that you welcome his or her advice while you are in the information-gathering phase.

Step 5. Visit the Web sites listed previously to review the information on the clinical trials that interest you. Each clinical trial that is listed will usually have the following components: the clinical trial objective, in other words, what the scientists are trying to learn from conducting the clinical trial; where the clinical trial will be conducted; and the patient eligibility criteria. Patient eligibility criteria are used to select which patients will be in the clinical trial; examples of criteria are age, extent of disease involvement, or the amount of prior treatment the patient has received.

Step 6. Compare the clinical trial eligibility criteria you found on the Web page or discussed with a clinical trial telephone service with your diagnosis and then select the clinical trials you think might be a match. Review these trials with your doctor, your family, and head and neck cancer survivors to get their opinions.

Before you seek your doctor's advice, try to narrow the selection down to two or three clinical trials. It is important to avoid presenting your doctor with a huge stack of clinical trials. If you need help in narrowing the choice, patient advocacy organizations can assist you, or you can call 800-4-CANCER.

Selecting the Clinical Trial That Is Right for You

Step 1. Determine how far are you willing to travel from your home to participate in a clinical trial.

Step 2. Locate the phone number of the clinical trial site where you are interested in participating. Sometimes the phone number that is listed is the clinical trial site and sometimes it is an 800 number to a service providing the clinical trial information to callers. Telephone numbers can be found on the clinical trial listing.

Step 3. Review the clinical trial eligibility criteria. If you think you may be eligible to enter the clinical trial, call the clinical trial site to determine whether you are in fact eligible for the clinical trial. Your doctor can call the clinical trial site for you, but that may not be necessary. At some point, the clinical trial site may want to speak to your doctor, but while you are in the process of gathering information, it usually is not necessary.

Step 4. Ask to speak to the protocol nurse or research assistant when you reach the clinical trial site. The phone number listed for the clinical trial is that of the physician who is also known as the principal investigator of the clinical trial. You are only gathering information, so it is not necessary to speak to this physician. Eventually, your doctor will speak to the principal investigator, but only when you decide to enter the clinical trial.

Step 5. Ask the following questions when speaking with the research assistant or protocol nurse:

■ Is the clinical trial still recruiting patients? If the clinical trial is no longer recruiting patients, the rest of the questions are irrelevant. Keep in mind that the database information sometimes lags behind the actual status of a clinical trial. For example, a clinical trial may be listed as open and recruiting patients but may actually have closed and the database has not yet been updated to reflect that fact.

■ Am I eligible for the clinical trial? This is the point when you recount a brief summary of your history, for example, the exact diagnosis, cell type, stage of disease, your age, and so on.

■ What is the objective of the clinical trial?

■ How may patients have been recruited so far? How many more will be recruited?

■ Can I get a copy of the informed consent document?

Step 6. Express your interest in entering the clinical trial if is still recruiting, but consult your family, your physician, and your patient advocacy organization before making your final decision. Remember that there are a many points of view concerning clinical trials. Deciding to participate is your decision.

Following are some additional questions to consider in your decision-making process:

■ Will my health insurance pay for my care if I enter a clinical trial?

■ Should I do it if my doctor disagrees?

■ Will placebos (inactive pill, liquid, or powder that has no treatment value) be used and why? Will study subjects receiving the placebo be offered the study drug after the comparative part of the study is completed?

■ What support is offered to patients in the clinical trial? For example, are travel expenses reimbursed?

■ Can I trust Web site information?

Finding a clinical trial to meet your needs is a complex process. However, there are many experienced cancer survivors waiting and willing to help you. The staff at the FDA's Cancer Liaison Program (301-796-8460 or http://www.fda.gov/OSHI) and members of the National Survivor Volunteer Network of SPOHNC are available to assist you.

Accessing Investigational Drugs Outside of a Clinical Trial

Most use of investigational medical treatments occurs in clinical trials. Clinical trials generally have inclusionary and exclusionary criteria for entry. Sometimes patients do not qualify for entry into a clinical trial, cannot travel to study sites, or they may wish to receive treatment with investigational drugs outside a clinical trial.

Expanded access, sometimes called "compassionate use," is the use of an investigational drug outside of a clinical trial to treat a patient with a serious or immediately life-threatening disease or condition who has no comparable or satisfactory alternative treatment options.

FDA regulations allow access to investigational drugs for treatment purposes on: (1) a case-by-case basis for an individual patient through a single patient investigational new drug (IND) application, (2) for many patients with similar treatment needs who otherwise do not qualify to participate in a clinical trial through a treatment IND, and (3) for an individual patient with a medical emergency through an emergency IND.

In order for a patient to gain access to an investigational drug outside of a clinical trial: (1) the patient must have a serious or immediately life-threatening disease or condition and no comparable or satisfactory therapeutic alternatives, (2) the patient must be ineligible or unable to participate in a clinical trial for the drug, (3) the manufacturer must be willing to provide the drug for treatment, and (4) the patient's physician must be willing to administer the drug and assume responsibility for the patient's care. If these four conditions are met, the manufacturer and the patient's doctor must make special arrangements to obtain the drug for the patient. These arrangements must be authorized by the FDA.

Because the drug is investigational, a review of the protocol by an Institutional Review Board (IRB) and an informed consent are required. These safeguards are in place to avoid exposing patients to unnecessary risks.

Sometimes, it is not possible for a patient to access an investigational drug outside a clinical trial. Manufacturers may not always be willing or able to provide access to a drug outside of their clinical trials, and they are not required to make their drug available through expanded access, or to make more of a drug for that purpose. Physicians may not always be able to seek expanded access for patients, depending on a patient's medical history and the risks associated with taking an investigational drug. The physician must determine that the probable risk from the drug is not greater than the probable risk from the disease. Not all physicians are willing to manage the use of an investigational drug for patients in their care. And, finally, even when an expanded access program has been established, sometimes there may not be enough of a drug available for all patients requesting access. Some companies establish lotteries to determine which patients will have treatment access, while others make the determination on a case-by-case basis.

Some but not all expanded access programs are listed on http://www.clinicaltrials.gov. However, even if a drug is not listed, you can still submit a request to obtain access to the drug. Your doctor will need to contact the drug manufacturer to determine whether they are willing and able to make the drug available. If they are willing to make the treatment available, it may or may not be necessary for your doctor to contact FDA to determine whether the treatment is eligible for expanded access for your disease. If you are interested in seeking expanded access to an investigational drug product, you or your healthcare professional can get information about the application process at http://www .fda.gov/Drugs/DevelopmentApprovalProcess/HowDrugsare DevelopedandApproved/ApprovalApplications/Investigational NewDrugINDApplication/ucm107434.htm. For additional information and assistance, contact the staff of FDA's Cancer Liaison Program (301-796-8460 or http://www.fda.gov/OSHI).

16

PRODUCTS, THERAPIES, AND SURVIVOR INPUT: RESOURCES FOR COPING WITH THE CHALLENGES OF SIDE EFFECTS OF TREATMENT

Compiled by Nancy E. Leupold, MA

Oral and head and neck cancer and its treatments can cause various side effects during a survivor's cancer journey. Some of these side effects can be easily controlled; others may require special types of care. The following tables have been compiled to provide information and supportive care to oral and head and neck cancer survivors who may be experiencing side effects of cancer and its treatment. It is important to keep in mind that not all survivors will experience the same side effects and not all suggested resources will be of help to everyone.

For information concerning the challenges of eating and swallowing and nutrition, please see Chapters 12 and 13 in this book.

DISCLAIMER: Support for People with Oral and Head and Neck Cancer (SPOHNC) does not endorse any treatments or products mentioned in this chapter. *It is of utmost importance that you consult with your physician and other health care professionals before using any of the treatments, products, tips, or suggestions presented on the following pages.*

Xerostomia (Dry Mouth) Saliva Substitutes

Product	Source	Description	How to Access
Chloraseptic Sore Throat Relief	Prestige Brands Inc. Survivor Input	Chloraseptic lozenges and sprays provide relief of sore throat pain and irritation. Assorted Flavors. Also available as diabetic-friendly, sugar-free solution.	Pharmacies. Supermarkets. Convenience stores http://www.chloraseptic.com
Entertainer's Secret Throat Relief Spray	KLI Corp.	Moisturizes, soothes, lubricates, mends and protects sensitive mucous membranes of the throat and larynx. A spray for dry sore throat and hoarse voice. Available in handy pocket/lipstick size	800-308-7452. http://www.entertainers-secret.com
MEDActive Oral Relief Gel	MedActive, LLC	Stimulates and enhances saliva flow. Contains ULTRAMULSION, a patented saliva soluble coating. Relieves burning sensations. No prescription necessary. This product is alcohol and sugar free, orange-crème flavor.	866-887-4867 http://www.medactive.com
MEDActive Oral Relief Lozenges	MedActive, LC	Formulated to relieve the discomfort of Dry Mouth (Xerostomia) and Sjögren's syndrome. They are the only lozenges to combine ULTRAMULSION, Spilanthes extract, and Pectin, creating a great tasting, long-lasting mouth feel experience that relieves the discomfort associated with insufficient saliva production.	866-887-4867 http://www.medactive.com

continues

Xerostomia (Dry Mouth) Saliva Substitutes *continued*

Product	Source	Description	How to Access
MED*Active* Patient-Friendly™ Oral Relief Spray	MedActive, LLC	Lubricates oral tissues and helps replenish saliva. Relieves burning sensations. Alcohol-free and sugar-free.	866-887-4867 http://www.medactivecom
MED*Active* Patient Friendly Oral Rinse	MedActive, LLC	Delivers 0.63% Stannous Fluoride, ULTRAMULSION, and natural Spilanthes extract to clean, lubricate, moisten, and protect the entire mouth.	866-887-4867 http//:www.medactive.com
Moi-stir	Kingswood Laboratories, Inc.	Moisturizes and lubricates oral tissues. Available in 4-oz. and 1-oz. sizes	Ask pharmacist to order 800-968-7772. http://www.kingswood-labs.com
Mouth Kote Dry Mouth Spray	Parnell Pharmaceuticals	Moisturizes mouth. Oral moisturizer with Yerba Santa. Contains xylitol. No sugar or alcohol. 2 oz. and 8 oz. sprays	Ask pharmacist to order or call 800-457-4276 http://www.parnellpharm.com
Numoisyn Liquid	Align Pharmaceuticals	Used to replace saliva when salivary glands are damaged. An oral solution with a viscosity similar to that of natural saliva.	**Consult your physician. By prescription only.** 908-834-0960 http://www.alignpharma.com

Product	Source	Description	How to Access
Numoisyn Lozenges	Align Pharmaceuticals	Increases salivary secretion by stimulating gustatory (taste) pathways. Lozenges.	**Consult your physician. By prescription only.** 908-834-0960 http://www.alignpharma.com
Oasis Moisturizing Mouthwash	Oasis Consumer Healthcare	Moisturizes mouth. Locks in moisture. Protects from dryness.	Pharmacies. Online stores. 888-936-2747 http://www.oasisdrymouth .com
Oasis Moisturizing Mouth Spray	Oasis Consumer Healthcare	Moisturizes mouth. Locks in moisture. Protects from dryness. Sugar-free, alcohol-free.	Pharmacies. Online stores. 888-936-2747 http://www.oasisdrymouth .com
Oral Balance Gel	GlaxoSmithKline Consumer Healthcare, L.P. (GSK)	Soothes and protects oral tissues. Antibacterial moisturizing gel.	Pharmacies. Online stores. 800-922-5856 http://www.biotene.com
Oral Balance Liquid	GlaxoSmithKline Consumer Healthcare, L.P. (GSK)	Helps promote healing as it moistens. Helpful in relieving severe dry mouth symptoms: burning, sore tissues, cotton palate, and swallowing difficulties.	Pharmacies. Online stores. 800-922-5856 http://www.biotene.com

continues

Xerostomia (Dry Mouth) Saliva Substitutes *continued*

Product	Source	Description	How to Access
Oral Balance Spray	GlaxoSmithKline Consumer Healthcare, L.P. (GSK)	Moisturizes mouth. Soothes and relieves dryness. Contains 5 moisturizers, 18 amino acids, calcium, and omega-3.	Pharmacies. Online stores. 800-922-5856 http://www.biotene.com
OraMoist Dry Mouth Disc	Quantum Health	Adheres to the roof of the mouth and moisturizes for up to 4 hours. Developed to alleviate parched, dry mouth.	Online stores. 800-448-1448 http://www.quantumhealth.com
QuenchMist Mouth Spray	Mueller Sports Medicine Inc.	Moisturizes mouth. Spray. Lemon, orange, cherry, and grape flavors.	Sporting goods store 800-356-9522 http://www.quenchgum.com.
Stoppers 4 Dry Mouth Spray	Woodridge Labs Inc.	Moisturizes mouth. Multiple enzyme formulation to maintain optimum moisture levels.	Pharmacies. Online stores. 888-766-7331 http://www.woodridgelab.com
THAYERS Sugar-free Dry Mouth Spray	Thayers Natural Remedies	Provides saliva-replacing moisture and instant relief from dryness. All natural, sugar-free. Peppermint and Citrus flavors.	Health food stores. 888-842-9371 http://www.thayers.com
Water, a survivor's best friend	Survivor input	Moisturizes the mouth. No sugar or salt. Available in many sizes and containers.	Pharmacies. Supermarkets. Homes.

Product	Source	Description	How to Access
XEROSDry Mouth Pump	CranioMandibular Rehab, Inc.	Portable saliva replacement system for patients with chronic dry mouth or xerostomia. Pumps any fluid from a reservoir into a foam mouthpiece at user-set intervals, as needed for comfort.	Online stores. 800-206-8381 http://www.Craniorehab.com

Xerostomia (Dry Mouth): Products and Therapies to Stimulate Salivary Flow
(Some products for dry mouth may "sting" on contact, but "stinging" usually disappears.)

Product	Distributor	Description	How to Access
Acupuncture	Survivor input	May be helpful in stimulating salivary glands to produce saliva.	**Consult your physician.** 510-649-8488 http://www.hmieducation.com
Biotēne Dry Mouth Gum	GlaxoSmithKline Consumer Healthcare, L.P. (GSK)	Stimulates salivary flow. Antibacterial. Sugar free. Reduces mouth sugars. Doesn't stick to dentures.	Pharmacies. 800-922-5856 http://www.bioteen.com
Carefree Sugarless Gum	Nabisco Inc.	Helps to stimulate saliva flow. Sugarless gum. Natural and artificial sweeteners. Assorted flavors.	Pharmacies. Supermarkets. Convenience stores. 312-644-2121

continues

Xerostomia (Dry Mouth): Products and Therapies to Stimulate Salivary Flow *continued*

Product	Distributor	Description	How to Access
Evoxac (Cevimeline HCl)	Daiichi Pharmaceuticals	Stimulates salivary glands to produce more saliva. Capsules. Not presently approved for head and neck cancer patients.	**Consult your physician. By prescription only.** http://www.evoxac.com
Extra™ Sugar-Free Gum	Wm. Wrigley Jr. Company	Stimulates saliva flow. Sugar-free gum sweetened with sorbitol, mannitol, and aspartame. Assorted natural and artificial flavors.	Pharmacies. Supermarkets. Convenience stores. http://www.wrigley.com
Fruit pits: peach, cherry, plum, etc.	Survivor Input	Sucking on fruit pit may stimulate salivary flow.	Supermarkets. Farm stands.
Hersheys IceBreakers	The Hershey Company Survivor Input	Refreshes the mouth with crisp flavor crystals. Provides a cooling sensation. Sweetened with sorbital. Available as mints and gum. Several flavors.	Pharmacies. Target, Supermarkets 800-468-1714 http://www.hersheys.com
Maxisal	Amarillo Biosciences Inc.	A dietary supplement containing Salive. Enhances salivary function. Promotes oral comfort. Helps relieve dry mouth.	Specific pharmacies 806-376-1741 http://www.amarbio.com
Salagen (pilocarpine HCL)	MGI Pharma Inc.	Stimulates the salivary glands to increase production of saliva. Tablets. 5,g and 7.5 mg.	**Consult your physician. By prescription only.** 800-562-0679

Product	Distributor	Description	How to Access
SalivaSure	Scandinavian Formulas, Inc.	Increases saliva production through the physiologic stimulation of taste buds. Self-dissolving lozenges provide instant relief for dry mouth upon contact.	Online stores. 800-688-2276 http://www .scandinavianformulas.com
Spry Rain Dry Mouth Spray	Xlear, Inc.	Provides immediate relief to dry mouth conditions with safe and effective xylitol. Has moisturizing effects and encourages increased salivation. Natural spearmint flavor.	Online stores. Health food stores 877-599-5327 http://www.xlear.com
THAYERS Sugar Free Dry Mouth Lozenges	Henry Thayer & Company	Stimulates saliva flow providing relief from dryness. All natural. Sugar-free.	Health food stores. Whole foods. 888-842-9371 http://www.thayers.com
THAYERS Sugar-Free Dry Mouth Spray	Henry Thayer & Company	Delivers soothing, natural, instant moisture and relief from dry mouth	Health food stores. Whole foods. 888-842-9371 http://www.thayers.com
TheraGum	Omni 3M ESPE	Stimulates saliva flow. Strengthens teeth. May reduce caries. Aids in reducing plaque. Promotes neutral pH. 100% xylitol.	Available in dental offices. http://www.4oralcare.com

continues

Xerostomia (Dry Mouth): Products and Therapies to Stimulate Salivary Flow *continued*

Product	Distributor	Description	How to Access
Theramints 100% Xylitol Lozenges	3M ESPW	Aid in reducing plaque, stimulate saliva flow to fight the harmful effects of dry mouth. Come in great fruit tasting flavors.	Online stores 888-364-3577 http://www.shop3m.com
Trident Gum	Cadbury Adams	Stimulates saliva flow. Sugarless chewing gum. Many flavors sweetened with xylitol.	Pharmacies. Supermarkets. Convenience stores.

Products to Help With Thick Saliva

Product	Source	Description	How to Access
Adolph's meat tenderizer	Survivor input	May help to break up thick saliva. 1 teaspoon tenderizer in 1 cup water. Swish and gargle but do not swallow. Do not use if there are open lesions in the mouth.	Online stores. Supermarkets. http://www.amazon.com
Bed wedge	Survivor input	Elevates head and supports the back and torso on a gradual slope. Available in different heights.	Medical supply companies. Online stores.
Blocks of wood under head of bed	Survivor input	Elevates the head.	Home Depot. Lowe's. Local lumberyard.

Product	Source	Description	How to Access
Ginger ale	Survivor input	Helps to clear mucus and reduce mucous-induced nausea	Supermarkets. Convenience stores.
Ginger tea (decaffeinated)	Survivor input	Sipping ginger tea may help to break up thick saliva.	Health food stores. Online stores.
Mucinex Tablets (guaifenesin) Time-released.	Adams Laboratories Survivor input	Helps loosen phlegm (mucus) and thin bronchial secretions to rid the bronchial passageways of bothersome mucus and make coughs more productive. An expectorant.	**Consult your physician.** Pharmacies. Supermarkets. 1-866-MUCINEX http://www.mucinex.com
Oral suction machine	Various medical equipment companies	Used to physically remove secretions from the mouth and throat. This will allow a person to breathe, eat, and talk more comfortably.	**Consult your physician.**
Papaya juice (100% pure)	Survivor input	Swish and swallow papaya juice from a glass. May help to cut thick saliva. Do not use if there are open lesions in the mouth.	Online stores. Supermarkets. Health food stores.
Papaya juice and club soda or seltzer	Survivor input	Sip slowly from a glass to help cut thick saliva. Do not use if there are open lesions in the mouth	Online stores. Supermarkets. Convenience stores. Health food stores.

continues

Products to Help With Thick Saliva *continued*

Product	Source	Description	How to Access
Robitussin (guaifenesin)	Pfizer Survivor input	Helps to thin mucus and makes it easier to cough it up. An expectorant.	**Consult your physician** Pharmacies. Supermarkets.
Room humidifier (cool mist)	Survivor input	May help to thin secretions. Use to moisten room air, especially at night. Must be routinely cleaned to avoid mold contamination.	Department stores. Pharmacies. Medical supply stores. Online stores.
Seltzer (unflavored)	Survivor input	Sip or gargle and drink to help cut thick saliva.	Supermarkets. Convenience stores.

Products to Soothe the Oral Mucosa

Product	Source	Description	How to Access
Acidophilus	Survivor input	Can help restore normal bacterial flora in the body. May be helpful in the treatment of thrush. Probiotic, also called "friendly bacteria" or "good bacteria." Capsules or liquid.	Health food stores.
Aloe Vera juice	Survivor input	Helps with healing mouth sores. Swish; hold in mouth; spit out.	Health food stores.

Product	Source	Description	How to Access
Caphosol	EUSA Pharma	Provides soothing relief of oral throat. A mouth rinse to moisten, lubricate, and clean the oral cavity and mucosa of the mouth, tongue, and throat.	**Consult your physician. By prescription only.** 800-833-3533
Diflucan (fluconazole)	Pfizer, Inc.	Used to treat fungal infections, including yeast infections of the mouth, throat, esophagus, and other organs. Slows the growth of fungi.	**Consult your physician. By prescription only.** 800-438-1985
GelClair	EKR Therapeutics	Provides relief of pain from mucositis by adhering to the mucosal surface of the mouth. Soothes oral lesions of various etiologies. A bio-adherent oral gel.	**Consult your physician. By prescription only.** 877-207-5802
GUM Chlorhexidine Gluconate Oral Rinse USP, 0.12%	Sunstar Americas Inc.	Helps fight bacteria, viruses, bacterial spores and fungi. Anti-microbial oral rinse. Alcohol-free. Therapeutically equivalent to Peridex.	**Consult your dentist.** 888-777-3101
Gum Rincinol P.R.N. Soothing Oral Rinse	Sunstar Americas, Inc.	Forms a protective barrier promoting healing of canker and mouth sores. No numbing benzocaine—No stinging hydrogen peroxide—No burning alcohol!	Pharmacies. 888-777-3101 http://www.drugstore.com

continues

Products to Soothe the Oral Mucosa *continued*

Product	Source	Description	How to Access
HurriCaine spray, liquid, or gel	Beutlich, LP, Pharmaceuticals	Relieves pain temporarily. Topical anesthetic containing 20% benzocaine. Several flavors.	Pharmacies. 800-238-8542 http://www.beutlich.com
Kefir	Survivor input	Swish and swallow. Pro-biotic dairy product that may restore oral flora.	Health food stores.
Kepivance (palifermin)	Biovitrum Survivor Input	Helps to decrease the incidence and duration of oral mucositis. Palifermin has not yet been approved for head and neck cancer patients.	**Consult your physician. By prescription only.** 866-773-5274 http://www.kepivance.com
Mary's Magic Mouthwash	Survivor input	Helps to relieve oral pain. A compound containing benadryl, an antiseptic, an antibiotic, and pain reliever. Swish and spit.	**Consult your physician. By prescription only.**
Mouthwash	Survivor input	Helps relieve pain due to oral ulcerations, Compound of Benadryl elixir, Maalox, Mylanta, or Kaopectate. Swish and spit.	**Consult your physician. By prescription only.**
Mouth Rinse (baking soda and salt)	Survivor input	Helps to relieve pain. Mix ½ teaspoon baking powder and ½ teaspoon salt with 1 quart warm water. Swish and spit out. Rinse with water.	**Consult your physician.** Ingredients available at supermarkets.

Product	Source	Description	How to Access
MuGard	Access Pharmaceuticals, Inc.	Ready-to-use rinse providing a protective coating to the oral mucosa for the treatment of mucositis.	**Consult your physician.** **By prescription only.** 214-905-5100 http://www.accesspharma .com
Mycelex® lozenge (clotrimazole)	Ortho-McNeil Pharmaceutical	Used to treat yeast infections of the mouth. Anti-fungal medication.	**Consult your physician.** **By prescription only.** 800-682-6532
Mycostatin (nystatin rinse)	Bristol-Myers Squibb company	Helps to treat thrush/candidacies. Swish, gargle, spit. Liquid, powder, lozenge.	**Consult your physician.** **By prescription only.** 800 321-1335
Peridex (chlorhexidine gluconate, 0.12%)	3M ESPE	Helps to fight bacteria, viruses, bacterial spores and fungi. An antiseptic and disinfectant antimicrobial. May help to prevent candidiasis.	**By prescription only** **Dental offices.** 800-634-2249
Prevention Antibacterial Mouth Rinse	Prevention Laboratories, LLC	Fights plaque and gingivitis. Kills bacteria; fights herpes virus and thrush. Helps heal mouth sores. Zinc/Hydrogen Peroxide. Alcohol free formula.	Walgreen's Pharmacy. Online stores 800-473-1205 http://www.preventionlab .com

continues

Products to Soothe the Oral Mucosa *continued*

Product	Source	Description	How to Access
Prevention Oncology Mouth Rinse	Prevention Laboratories, LLC	Soothes the oral tissues. Helps control sore gums and ulcerated tissue. Controls thrush. Alcohol-free.	Walgreen's Pharmacy. Online Stores. 800-473-1205 http://www.preventionlab.com
reBalance Ca	Vaxco Pharmaceuticals	Helps relieve the pain caused by oral mucositis.	913-236-6518 http://www.vaxcopharma.com
Sporanox (itraconazole)	Ortho-McNeil, Inc.	Used to treat yeast infections of the mouth and throat. Also used to treat fungal infections of the fingernails and/or toenails	**Consult your physician. By prescription only.** 800-526-7736
Tea tree oil (diluted)	Survivor input	May be helpful for the treatment of thrush. Tea tree oil is known as an effective antiseptic and fungicide. Promotes tissue healing.	**Consult your physician.** Health food stores.
THAYERS Slippery Elm Lozenges	Henry Thayer and Company	Soothes the tissues of the mouth and throat. All natural, sugar free lozenges. Several flavors available.	Health food stores. 888-842-9371 http://www.thayers.com

Product	Source	Description	How to Access
Toothette Oral Care Mouth Moisturizer	Sage Products, Inc.	Soothes and moisturizes lips and oral tissues with vitamin E and coconut oil.	Ask your pharmacist to order. Sage Products, Inc. 800-323-2220 http://www.sageproducts.com
Toothette Swabs	Sage Products, Inc.	Cleans teeth and soothes mouth. Various swabs available.	Ask your pharmacist to order. Sage Products, Inc. 800-323-2220 http://www.sageproducts.com
UlcerEase	Med-Derm Pharmaceuticals	Helps to relieve pain due to mouth ulcers, canker sores and other irritations. Sodium bicarbonate based alcohol-free anesthetic mouth rinse.	Pharmacies. 800-877-8869 http://www.crown laboratories.com http://www.drugstore.com
Xylocaine Viscous (lidocaine viscous)	AstraZeneca Pharmaceuticals	May help to relieve pain associated with radiation mucositis. Topical anesthetic.	**Consult your physician. By prescription only.** 800-236-9933

251

Products to Soothe the Nasal Passages

Product	Source	Description	How to Access
Advil Congestion Relief	Pfizer	Combines the power of Advil plus an effective decongestant to relieve sinus pressure, nasal swelling and congestion and headache.	Pharmacies. Online stores. 800-882-3845 http://www.advil.com
Alkalol	The Alkalol Company (Survivor Input)	Helps dissolve mucus and clear blocked nasal passages. A unique blend of natural ingredients	Pharmacies. Online stores. 800-967-4904 http://www.alkalolcompany.com.
Ayr Saline Nasal Gel Moisturizing Swabs	B. F. Ascher and Co.	Helps moisturize and soothe dry noses.	Pharmacies. Online stores. 913-888-1880 http://www.drugstore.com
Ayr Saline Nasal Gel with Soothing Aloe	B. F. Ascher and Co.	Moisturizes and soothes dry, stuffy sore, tender noses.	Pharmacies. Online Stores. 913-888-1880 http://www.drugstore.com
Ayr Saline Nasal Mist	B. F. Ascher and Co	Moisturizes nasal passages relieving dry, crusty and inflamed nasal membranes	Pharmacies. Online Stores. 913-888-1880 http://www.drugstore.com

Product	Source	Description	How to Access
Homemade rinse	Survivor input	Helps relieve stuffiness and blockage. ½ tsp salt, ½ tsp baking soda mixed in warm water. Use nasal irrigator syringe to administer.	**Consult your physician.** Supermarket for ingredients.
NeilMed Sinus Rinse	NeilMed Pharmaceuticals	Helps relieve stuffiness and blockage of the nasal passages. A therapeutic, saline nasal irrigation & moisturizing system.	Pharmacies. Online stores. 877-477-8633 http://www.neilmed.com
Pretz Concentrate	Parnell Pharmaceuticals	Used for moisturizing the nasal mucosa and sinuses. Preservative free with Yerba Santa and xylitol. Mix with water.	800-457-4276 http://www.parnellpharm.com http://www.yslabs.com
Pretz Irrigation	Parnell Pharmaceuticals	Provides moisturizing nasal irrigation with natural Yerba Santa.	800-457-4276 http://www.parnellpharm.com http://www.yslabs.com
Pretz Spray	Parnell Pharmaceuticals	Used for moisturizing the nasal mucosa and sinuses. 3% glycerin in saline nasal spray with Yerba Santa.	800-457-4276 http://www.parnellpharm.com http://www.yslabs.com
Simply Saline Nasal Mist	Church & Dwight Co., Inc.	Helps clear congestion, dust and debris while improving the ability to smell and gain clearer breathing. Purified water, 0.9% Sodium Chloride	Pharmacies. Online stores. 800-524-1328 http://www.churchdwight.com http://www.SimplySaline.com

Products to Help Trismus (A restriction in the opening of the mouth)

Product	Source	Description	How to Access
Botox	Allergan Inc.	Decreases spasms of jaw muscles. Local injection.	**Consult your physician. By prescription only.** 800-377-7790
Dynasplint Trismus System	Dynasplint Systems Inc.	Aids in restoring range of motion to tight and short jaw muscles that cause restricted mouth opening.	800-638-6771 http://www.dynasplint.com
TheraBite Jaw Motion Rehabilitation System™	Atos Medical	Designed to treat trismus, limited jaw mobility and orofacial pain. Utilizes repetitive passive motion and stretching to restore mobility and flexibility of jaw musculature, associated joints, and connective tissues.	Consult insurance company for preauthorization. 877-458-ATOS (2867) or 800-217-0025 http://www.atosdirect.com
TheraJaw Hot/Cold Cooler System	CranioMandibular Rehab, Inc.	Continually treats swelling and pain in face and jaw by pumping hot or cold water through pads on the face. Lasts 4–8 hours. May be rented or purchased.	1-800-206-8381 http://www.craniorehab.com
OraStretch press jaw motion rehab system	CranioMandibular Rehab, Inc.	A jaw stretching device for preventing and treating trismus from surgery, radiation or joint dysfunction.	Consult insurance company for preauthorization. Online stores 800-206-8381 http://www.craniorehab.com

Products for Oral Hygiene
(Toothpaste)

Product	Source	Description	How to Access
Aquafresh Toothpaste	GlaxoSmithKline (GSK)	Fluoride toothpaste for cavity protection. Tubes and pumps.	Pharmacies. Supermarkets. 800-897-5623 http://www.aquafresh.com
Biotene Dry Mouth Denture Grip	GlaxoSmithKline Consumer Healthcare, L.P. (GSK)	Formulated to provide a strong, long-lasting and comfortable hold in a dry mouth. Soothes minor irritations. Refreshing taste.	Pharmacies. Online stores. 800-922-5856 http://www.biotene.net
Biotene Dry Mouth Toothpaste	GlaxoSmithKline Consumer Healthcare, L.P. (GSK)	Contains antibacterial enzymes to destroy bacteria. Helps restore natural antibacterial system present in saliva. Contains fluoride. 4.5 oz. tube.	Pharmacies. 800-922-5856 http://www.biotene.net
Clinpro 5000 1.1% Sodium Fluoride Anti-Cavity Toothpaste	3M ESPE	Contains fluoride as well as calcium and phosphate, which are components naturally found in saliva.	800-634-2249 http://www.3mesps.com
PreviDent 5000 Plus toothpaste	Colgate Oral Pharmaceuticals	Used to help prevent cavities. Prescription-strength fluoride treatment	**Dental offices only. By prescription only.** 800-643-3639 http://www.colgate.com

continues

255

Products for Oral Hygiene (Toothpaste) *continued*

Product	Source	Description	How to Access
Tom's of Maine Children's Toothpaste	Tom's of Maine Survivor Input	Only natural kid's toothpaste to earn the ADA Seal of Acceptance. That means proven effective, cavity fighting protection. Doesn't burn your mouth.	Pharmacies. Supermarkets. Online stores. 800-367-8667 http://www.tomsofmaine.com
Tom's of Maine Dry Mouth Anti-Cavity Fluoride Toothpaste	Tom's of Maine	Aids in the prevention of dental cavities. Contains xylitol. Mild apricot or strawberry flavor.	Pharmacies, Supermarkets. Online stores. 800-367-8667

(Toothbrushes, etc.)

Product	Source	Description	How to Access
Biotene Super Soft Toothbrush	GlaxoSmithKline Consumer Healthcare, L.P. (GSK)	Ensures a gentle cleaning without irritating inflamed or unhealthy tissues.	Pharmacies. Online stores. 800-922-5856 http://www.biotene.net
Dental Water Jet	Many manufacturers Survivor Input	Helps people with dry mouth to clear debris after eating and before brushing teeth.	Pharmacies. Department stores. Online stores.

Product	Source	Description	How to Access
Oral-B Pro-Health Gentle Clean Toothbrush	Procter & Gamble	Provides gentle cleaning. Extra soft brush, with extra soft CrissCross bristles	Pharmacies. Supermarkets. Online stores. 800-566-7252 http://www.oralb.com
Plackers Gentle Fine Flosser	Placontrol, Inc. (Survivor input)	Allows for gentle flossing between back teeth when full opening of mouth is possible.	Pharmacies. Online stores. http://www.plackers.com
Rota-dent Electric Toothbrush	Zila Pharmaceuticals	Power-assisted rotary toothbrush. Soft filament brush tips.	**Dental offices only.** 800-752-2564
SensodyneTotal Care Toothbrush	GlaxoSmithKline (GSK)	Dome-shaped head designed to adapt to gum line. Extra soft, round-ended bristles to help prevent gum irritation.	Pharmacies. Online stores. 888-825-5249

(Mouthwash)

Product	Source	Description	How to Access
Biotene Mouthwash	GlaxoSmithKline Consumer Healthcare, L.P. (GSK)	Breaks down bacteria. Replaces important enzymes. Antibacterial enzyme system. Alcohol-free.	Pharmacies. 800-922-5856 http://www.biotene.net

continues

Products for Oral Hygiene (Mouthwash) *continued*

Product	Source	Description	How to Access
Biotene PBF Mouthwash	GlaxoSmithKline Consumer Healthcare, L.P. (GSK)	Formulated to remove and dissolve plaque and biofilm. Alcohol free. Kills germs more effectively. Fresh breath—6× longer	Pharmacies. 800-922-5856 http://www.biotene.net
Colgate Dry Mouth Relief Fluoride Mouthwash	Colgate Palmolive Company	Provides soothing relief. Contains fluoride to help reduce the risk of cavities. Alcohol-free. Moisturizing mint flavor. Available in 16 oz.	Pharmacies. Online stores.. 800-2265-6283 http://www.colgate professional.com
Orazyme-Dry Mouth Mouthwash	Dr. Fresh Inc.	Moistens the mouth on contact and lasts for hours. It soothes and protects irritated oral tissue and promotes healing of cracks and sores due to dry mouth conditions.	Online stores, only. 866-373-7374 http://www.orazyme.net
PerioMed Oral Rinse	Omnii Oral Pharmaceuticals 3M ESPE	Contains patented plaque fighter. Alcohol-free. Flavored base. Pump.	**Dental offices. By prescription only.** 800-634-2249
Perox-A-Mint Oral Solution Rinse	Sage Products Inc.	Mechanically cleans and debrides without drying. Mint flavored 1.5% hydrogen peroxide solution rinse	Online stores 800-323-2220 http://www.sageproducts.com

Product	Source	Description	How to Access
PreviDent Dental Rinse	Colgate Oral Pharmaceuticals	Used as a weekly dental rinse. Four times the fluoride of over-the-counter toothpastes.	**Dental offices.** **By prescription only.** 800-643-3639 http://www.colgate.com
SmartMouth Mouthwash	Triumph Pharmaceuticals	Effective for common and chronic bad breath. 100% alcohol-free, no burning. 2-bottle, 2-pump system.	Pharmacies. Supermarkets. http://www.drugstore.com
SootheRX	3M ESPE	Indicated for both the rapid and continual relief of dentinal hypersensitivity The first FDA cleared at-home prescription therapy	**Dental Offices.** 800-643-3639

Products to Protect Teeth

Product	Source	Description	How to Access
ACT Rinse	Johnson & Johnson	Anticavity fluoride rinse (0.05%). Alcohol-free and nonirritating. Use once daily after brushing.	Pharmacies. Online stores. 800-526-3967

continues

Products to Protect Teeth *continued*

Product	Source	Description	How to Access
Custom gel fluoride trays	Dental offices	Used to prevent demineralization of tooth structure and rampant caries. Best way to provide adequate fluoride.	**Consult your dentist. Dental offices.**
Gel Kam (0.4% stannous fluoride gel)	Colgate Oral Pharmaceuticals	Brush-on gel with 0.4% stannous fluoride for caries prevention and hypersensitivity relief.	Pharmacies. 800-468-6502 http://www.colgate.com
Gel-Kam Home Care Gel	Colgate Oral Pharmaceuticals	Provides sensitivity relief and cavity protection.	Pharmacies. 800-468-6502 http://www.colgate.com
Gel-Kam Oral Care Rinse	Colgate Oral Pharmaceuticals	Reduces existing plaque. High concentration of stannous fluoride for maximum sensitivity relief.	**Dental offices. By prescription only.** 800-468-6502 http://www.colgate.com
PerioMed (0.63% stannous fluoride oral rinse)	3M ESPE	Provides consistent stannous and fluoride ion bioavailability. Contains patented plaque fighter. Alcohol-free. Flavored base. Pump.	**Dental offices. By prescription only.** 800-643-3639

Product	Source	Description	How to Access
Omni Gel™ (0.4% stannous fluoride gel)	Omni Preventive Care, a 3M ESP Company	Provides caries reduction, enhanced remineralization. Brush-on gel. Assorted flavors.	**Dental offices.** **By prescription only.** 800-364-3577 http://www.3m.com
Oral B Minute Foam	Procter & Gamble Survivor Input	Provides protective fluoride to patients in formulas designed for safe, easy home use. Available in many flavors.	**Dental offices.** **By prescription only.** 1-800-566-7252
Phos-Flur Floride Gel	Colgate Oral Pharmaceuticals	Used frequently with custom mouth trays for daily self-topical use as a dental caries preventative. Promotes remineralization.	**Dental offices.** **By prescription only.** 800-643-3639 http://www.colgate.com
PreviDent Brush on Gel	Colgate Oral Pharmaceuticals	Used in a custom mouth tray. Five times the fluoride of over-the-counter toothpastes.	**Dental offices.** **By prescription only.** 800-643-3639 http://www.colgate.com

continues

261

Products to Protect Teeth *continued*

Product	Source	Description	How to Access
PreviDent Dental Rinse	Colgate Oral Pharmaceuticals	Used as a weekly dental rinse. Four times the fluoride of over-the-counter toothpastes.	**Dental offices.** **By prescription only.** 800-643-3639 http://www.colgate.com
Thera-Flur-N gel-drops	Novartis	Helps to prevent dental caries. Once-daily use. Self-applied topical brand of neutral sodium fluoride added	**Dental offices.** **By prescription only.**
Vanish 5% Sodium Fluoride White Varnish	3M Company ESPE	Provides enhanced flow characteristics for thorough coverage. Offers rapid set application time. Packaged as unit-doses. Contains xylitol. Available in cherry, melon, and mint flavors.	**Dental offices.** **By prescription only.** 800-364-3577 http://www.3m.com
Vanish XT	3M ESPE	Provides a protective barrier that immediately relieves sensitivity and provides a long-term release of fluoride, calcium and phosphate.	800-634-2249 http://www.3mespe.com

Products for Radiation Dermatitis

(Check with your radiation oncologist prior to radiation therapy to determine whether skin cream can be used prior to radiation or after radiation, only.)

Product	Source	Description	How to Access
Alra Therapy Lotion	Neue Cosmetic Company	Developed for the treatment of skin exposed to radiation therapy: Aloe vera gel, lanolin, vitamin E.	877-265-9092 http://www.alra.com http://www.healingbaskets .com
Aquaphor healing ointment	Eucerin Patient input	Reduces healing time. Creates protective barrier that seals in moisture. Helps heal raw, irritated skin caused by radiation treatments.	Pharmacies. Supermarkets. Online drug stores. http://www.eucerinus.com
Biafine	OrthoNeutrogena, Ortho-McNeil Pharmaceutical	Facilitates the recovery of compromised skin by impacting the three stages of healing. Provides moist environment for healing and repels harmful germs and other external contamination.	**Consult your physician. By prescription only.** 877-738-4624 http://www.orthoneutrogena .com
Baby Calendula Cream Nature's First Aid	Baby Survivor input	Used on extra-dry or sensitive skin. Botanically based, a light and fluffy calendula cream. Helps soothe radiated skin.	Whole Foods, Target, Babies R Us. Online stores. 877-576-2825 x 205 http://www.californiababy.com

continues

263

Products for Radiation Dermatitis *continued*

Product	Source	Description	How to Access
Elocon (mometasone furoate)	Merck	Used to relieve the redness, swelling, itching and discomfort of many skin problems. High potency topical corticosteroid. Cream, ointment, or lotion.	**Consult your physician. By prescription only.** 800-672-6372
Lindi Body Lotion	Lindi Skin	Helps to improve overall dryness resulting from chemotherapy. Light and refreshing.	800-380-4704 http://www.lindiskin.com Use online store locator
Lindi Cooler Roll	Lindi Skin	Provides immediate and cooling relief to burned or dehydrated skin. Use after each treatment.	800-380-4704 http://www.lindiskin.com Use online store locator
Lindi Skin Cooler Pad	Lindi Skin	Provides immediate and cooling relief to areas that are burned or dehydrated.	800-380-4704 http://www.lindiskin.com Use online store locator
Mepilex Border with Safetac soft silicone technology	Molnlyck Health Care	Used in the management of radiation skin reactions. Pad does not stick to moist wound bed. Absorbs moderate amounts of drainage. Adheres gently to surrounding dry skin.	Online stores. 800-843-8497 http://www.@molnlycke.com

Product	Source	Description	How to Access
Mepilex Lite with Safetac soft silicone technology	Molnlyck Health Care	Used in the management of radiation skin reactions. Thin, flexible, absorbent pad. Maintains a moist wound environment.	Online stores. 800-843-8497 http://www.@molnlycke.com
MepilexTransfer with Safetac soft silicone technology	Molnlyck Health Care	Used in the management of radiation skin reactions. A transfer dressing. Pad may be used as a protective layer on minimal or low oozing wounds.	Online stores. 800-843-8497 http://www.molnlycke.com
MPM CoolMagic Gel sheets	MPM Medical Inc.	Used to reduce pain from burns and skin reactions to radiation. Allows flow of oxygen. Prevents bacteria and foreign matter from entering the wound.	800-232-5512 http://www.mpmmedicalinc.com
Polysporin Ointment	Pfizer	Prevents infection to help speed healing.	Pharmacies. Supermarkets. 800-438-1985
RadiaCream Moisturizing Cream	Medline Industries	Used for moisturizing skin and post-healing in radiation patients. Softens and conditions rough, scaly skin.	Online stores. 800-633-5463
RadiaDresGel Sheet (4" × 4")	Medline Industries	Used in the management of partial thickness wounds relating to radiation-induced dermatitis.	Online stores. 800-633-5463

continues

265

Products for Radiation Dermatitis *continued*

Product	Source	Description	How to Access
RadiaGel Hydrogel wound dressing	Medline Industries	Can be used before, during, and after radiation. A hydrogel wound dressing with Acemannan Hydrogel. Provides soothing relief to radiation dermatitis.	Online stores. 800-633-5463
MPM RadiaPlexRx Gel	MPM Medical Inc.	Used to prevent and soothe skin problems associated with radiation dermatitis. A unique combination of complex carbohydrates and hyaluronic acid. Has ability to retain huge quantities of water.	**Consult your radiation oncologist.** **By prescription only.** Call 800-232-5512. http://www.mpmmedicalinc.com
Regenecare Wound Gel	MPM Medical Inc.	Used to reduce rash and itching. Reduces pain from radiation A pain-relieving hydrogel. Contains lidocaine HCl, collagen, and aloe vera.	**Consult your radiation oncologist.** **By prescription only.** Call 800-232-5512 http://www.mpmmedicalinc.com

Product	Source	Description	How to Access
Regenecare HA Wound Gel	MPM Medical Inc.	Used to reduce rash and itching. Reduces pain from radiation. A pain relieving hydrogel. Contains lidocaine HCl, collagen and aloe vera.	**Consult your radiation oncologist.** Call 800-232-5512 http://www.mpmmedicalinc .com
Remedy Repair Crème	Medline Industries Inc.	Helps restore natural moisture balance to skin while delivering vital nutrients. Moisturizes/protects skin.	Online stores. Pharmacies. 800-633-5463 http://www.medline.com
Siberian Seabuckthorn oil	Survivor input	Promotes healing of heat burns, radiation burns, sunburns, poorly healing wounds, bedsores, skin ulcers, and eczema.	Online stores.
Spand-Gel Wound Dressing	Medi-Tech International Corp.	Provides moist, cool wound-healing environment. Relieves pain, burning, itching, and soreness. Contains aloe vera. Available as a neck wrap.	Online stores. 800-333-0109 http://www.medi-techintl.com
Udderly Smooth Hand & Foot Cream	Redex Industries Inc.	Used to treat dry skin. Contains urea to enhance moisturizing. Smoothes roughness and softens skin. Unscented.	800-345-7339 http://www.udderlysmooth .com http://www.drugstore.com

continues

Products for Radiation Dermatitis *continued*

Product	Source	Description	How to Access
Vigilon Primary Wound Dressing	C. R. Bard Medical	Used on all partial and full thickness wounds (excluding 3rd degree burns). Ideal for skin tears, minor burns and radiation reactions.	Online stores. 800-526-4455 http://www.bardmedical.com
Vitamin E capsules and aloe vera gel	Patient input	Pierce a vitamin E capsule and apply contents to skin every night; remove before radiation treatments. Apply aloe vera on skin directly after treatment.	**Consult your radiation oncologist.** Pharmacies. Vitamin shops.
Xclair Cream	Align Pharmaceuticals	Increases hydration, reduces inflammation & soothes the skin damaged by radiation therapy. Does not contain steroids, immunomodulating substances, alcohol, or fragrance.	**Consult your physician. By prescription only.** 908-834-0960 http://www.align.com

Products and Therapies to Help Reduce Side Effects of Neck Dissections

Product	Source	Description	How to Access
Acupuncture	Survivor input	Used for the treatment of pain in the neck and shoulders resulting from neck dissection surgery.	**Consult your physician.**

Product	Source	Description	How to Access
Barnes Myofascial Release	Survivor input	Hands-on technique that provides sustained pressure into connective tissue to relieve pain and restore motion from tightness and restriction to the fascia caused by physical trauma, scarring, stress, and inflammation.	**Consult your physician. Consult a physical therapist.** http://www.myofascial release.com
Botox (botulinum toxin)	Allergan Inc.	Used to help stop muscle spasms. Injection.	**Consult your physician. By prescription only.**
Celebrex (celecoxib)	Pfizer	Used to relieve pain, tenderness, swelling, and stiffness.	**Consult your physician. By prescription only.** 800-438-1985
Physical therapy	Survivor input	For deep tissue release of muscle spasms and contracture of muscles.	**Consult your physician. Consult a physical therapist.**
Soma (carisoprodol)	MedPoint Pharmaceuticals	Relaxes muscles and relieves pain and discomfort. A muscle relaxant, used with rest, physical therapy, etc. May cause drowsiness.	**Consult your physician. By prescription only.** 888-766-2250
Trigger point massage therapy	Survivor input	Applies concentrated pressure to areas of chronic or severe pain in the muscles, called "trigger points." May help to free frozen shoulder.	**Consult your physician.** Consult a physical therapist.

Products to Help Relieve Lhermitte's Sign

(Electriclike shocks extending down the spine upon flexing the head caused by radiation toxicity to the central or peripheral nervous system)

Neuropathy

(Numbness, tingling sensation, muscle weakness, pain in the extremities)

Product	Source	Description	How to Access
Acupuncture	Survivor input	May help to reduce pain. Specific areas of the body are shallowly pierced with fine needles to relieve pain or produce regional anesthesia	**Consult your physician.** 510-649-8488 http://www.hmieducation.com
Elavil (amitriptyline)	Merck Sharp & Dohme Corp	Sometimes used to treat chronic pain. Also used in the treatment of Lhermitte's Sign at low doses. Considered a tricyclic antidepressant.	**Consult your physician.** **By prescription only.**
Lidoderm (lidocaine patch)	Endo Pharmaceuticals Inc.	Used to relieve pain. Class of medications called local anesthetics. Works by stopping nerves from sending pain signals.	**Consult your physician.** **By prescription only.**
Neurontin (gabapentin)	Pfizer	May help to relieve the pain of neuropathy and Lhermitte's sign at low doses. Class of medications called anticonvulsants. Tablet or liquid form.	**Consult your physician.** **By prescription only.** 800-438-1985

Product	Source	Description	How to Access
Tegreto (carbamazepine)	Novartis Pharmaceuticals	Used in the treatment of Lhermitte's sign at low doses. Tablet or liquid form. Anticonvulsant.	**Consult your physician.** **By prescription only.** 888-669-6682
Trental (pentoxifylline)	Sanofi-Aventis U.S. LLC Survivor Input	Used to improve blood flow in patients with circulation problems to reduce aching, cramping, and tiredness in the hands and feet. Survivor reports helping with blood flow to her tongue.	**Consult your physician.** **By prescription only.** 800-207-8049
Tofranil (imipramine)	Mallickrodt Inc.	Used in the treatment of Lhermitte's Sign at low doses. A tricyclic antidepressant. Tablet.	**Consult your physician.** **By prescription only.**
Transcutaneous electrical nerve stimulation (TENS)	TENS units made by different manufacturers	Works to decrease pain perception and may be used to control acute and chronic pain. Battery-operated stimulator.	**Consult your physician.** **Consult a physical therapist.** Online stores.

Products to Help Relieve Pain

Product	Source	Description	How to Access
Duragesic (fentanyl topical)	Janssen Pharmaceutical Products LP	Used to relieve pain. A narcotic (opioid) pain medicine. May cause drowsiness.	**Consult your physician. By prescription only.** 800-526-7736
Liquid Motrin (ibuprofen)	McNeil Consumer Healthcare	Used to help relieve pain. Easier to swallow than tablet.	Pharmacies. Supermarkets. 877-223-9807
Liquid Tylenol	McNeil Consumer Healthcare	Used to help relieve pain. Easier to swallow than tablet.	Pharmacies. Supermarkets. 877-223-9807
OxyContin (oxycodone)	Purdue Pharma	Used to relieve moderate to severe pain. May cause drowsiness. Liquid and tablet form.	**Consult your physician. By prescription only.** 888-726-7535
Prialt (ziconotide)	Elan Pharmaceuticals	Used to treat severe chronic pain. May cause drowsiness.	**Consult your physician. By prescription only.** 800-859-8586.
Therapeutic nerve blocks	Survivor input	Used to control pain. Nerve blocks contain local anesthetic. Injection.	**Consult your physician. By prescription only.**

Products and Therapies to Help Reduce Lymphedema

Product/Therapy	Description	How to Access
Compression bandaging	Used to treat lymphedema. Compression options may be difficult with facial edema. Bandage with short stretch bandages and sometimes combined with various types of foam. May help break up fibrosis in tissues as well as reduce the volume of edema.	**Consult your physician.** **Consult a physical therapist.** National Lymphedema Network 800-541-3259 http://www.lymphnet.org
Eucerin or Curél	Used to provide good skin care and hygiene to help avoid infections and wounds.	Pharmacies. Supermarkets 800-227-4703
Exercise	Used to improve biomechanical function and soften the tissues under the skin of the face and neck to reduce swelling. "Facial gymnastic exercises," deep breathing exercises. Pool exercise is excellent for lymphedema.	**Consult your physician.** **Consult a physical therapist.** National Lymphedema Network 800-541-3259 http://www.lymphet.org
Lymphedema alert bracelets	Used to provide awareness of lymphedema. Bracelets say: "Lymphedema Alert: No blood pressure and no needles into this arm."	National Lymphedema Network 800-541-3259 http://www.lymphnet.org

Products to Treat Anemia Caused by Poor Nutrition

Products	Description	How to Access
Cobalamin (vitamin B_{12})	Used in the treatment of pernicious anemia and anemia resulting from a lack of vitamin B_{12}. Given by injection.	**Consult your physician.** Pharmacies. Online stores.
Folic acid (B-complex vitamin)	Used for the treatment of folic acid deficiency anemia resulting from low levels of folic acid in the body caused by poor nutrition, poor absorption, and some medications.	**Consult your physician.** Pharmacies, health food stores.
Oral iron supplements (ferrous sulfate)	Used for iron deficiency anemia caused by too little iron in the diet, poor absorption of iron by the body, and gastrointestinal blood loss caused by ulcers and the use of aspirin and nonsteroidal anti-inflammatory medications (NSAIDS). Liquid prescriptions may stain teeth.	**Consult your physician.** Pharmacies, health food stores.

Products to Help With Chemotherapy-Induced Anemia

Product	Source	Description	How to Access
Aranesp (darbepoetin alfa)	Amgen	May be given as a series of injections to induce bone marrow to make more red blood cells.	**Consult your physician.** **By prescription only.**
Epogen (epoetin alfa)	Amgen	May be given as a series of injections to induce bone marrow to make more red blood cells.	**Consult your physician.** **By prescription only.**

Product	Source	Description	How to Access
Procrit (epoetin alfa)	Ortho Biotech Inc.	May be given as a series of injections to induce bone marrow to make more red blood cells.	**Consult your physician. By prescription only.**

Products to Help With Fatigue*

Product	Sources	Description	How to Access
Carnitor (levocarnitine)	Sigma-Tau Pharmaceuticals Patient input	Used to treat fatigue resulting from carnitine deficiency caused by chemotherapy or poor nutrition. Injection, capsules, or liquid.	**Consult your physician. By prescription only.** 800-447-0169
Provigil (modafinil)	Cephalon, Inc.	Improves wakefulness. May promote a sense of well-being, decreased fatigue, and increased appetite. Psychostimulant for cancer patients.	**Consult your physician. By prescription only.** 800-896-5855
Ritalin (methylphenidate hydrochloride)	Novartis Pharmaceuticals	May help cancer patients fight fatigue (otherwise used to treat attention deficit hyperactivity disorder in children).	**Consult your physician. By prescription only.** 888-669-6682
Synthroid (levothyroxine)	Abbott Laboratories	May help to decrease fatigue associated with reduced thyroid function.	**Consult your physician. By prescription only.**

*Treating anemia may also help fatigue.

Products to Help With Dehydration

Product	Source	Description	How to Access
Bouillon and broths	Many manufacturers	Provides hydration and electrolytes.	Supermarkets. Convenience stores. Online stores.
Gatorade	Gatorade Company	Provides essential hydration, salt replacement, and energy boost.	Pharmacies. Supermarkets. Online stores.
NutriSqueeze Dual Straw Pouch	CranioRehab.com	NutriSqueeze pouches are easy to use and can be taken anywhere. A great alternative to feeding syringes.	800-206-8381 http://www.craniorehab.com
NutriSqueeze bottles and syringes	CranioRehab.com	Helps decrease swelling and pain in face and jaw after surgery or radiation with soft hot/cold gel packs and compression.	800-206-8381 http://www.craniorehab.com
Pedialyte	Abbott Laboratories	Continually treats swelling and pain in face and jaw by pumping hot or cold water through pads on the face. Lasts 4–8 hours. Rented or purchased.	Pharmacies. Supermarkets. Convenience stores. Online stores.
Sports drinks: Powerade Accelerade Lucozade Sport	Many manufacturers	Helps to rehydrate and replenish electrolytes, sugar, water, and other nutrients.	Pharmacies. Supermarkets. Convenience stores. Online stores.

Products to Help With Nausea

Product	Source	Description	How to Access
Acupuncture	Survivor input	May help in the treatment of nausea.	**Consult your physician.** 510-649-8488 http://www.hmieducation.com
Compazine (prochlorperazine) (Generic now available,)	Many pharmaceutical companies	Used to treat nausea/vomiting. Tablet, extended release capsule, oral liquid, rectal suppository. May cause drowsiness.	**Consult your physician. By prescription only.** Online stores
Zofran	GlaxoSmithKline (GSK)	Used to prevent nausea and vomiting that may be caused by chemotherapy, radiation therapy, and surgery. Tablet and liquid.	**Consult your physician. By prescription only.** 888-825-5249

Products to Help Relieve Constipation

Product	Source	Description	How to Access
Aloe vera juice	Survivor input	Drink 3 to 4 mouthfuls at a time to help relieve constipation.	Health food stores.
Colace	Purdue Pharma LP	Indicated for the treatment of occasional constipation. Capsules, liquid, suppositories.	Pharmacies. Supermarkets. Online drugstores. 800-877-5666

continues

Products to Help Relieve Constipation *continued*

Product	Source	Description	How to Access
Dose of medication	Survivor input	Use of some medications may cause constipation. Dose may need to be adjusted.	**Consult your physician.**
Dulcolax (bisacodyl)	Boehringer Ingelheim Consumer Healthcare	Used on a short-term basis to treat constipation. Tablet, suppository.	Pharmacies. Supermarkets. 800-243-0127
Home remedy for bowel regularity	Survivor input	Mix ⅔ cup oat bran, ⅔ cup prune juice, and ⅔ cup unsweetened applesauce. Eat a few tablespoons to ½ cup, twice daily. Refrigerate unused portion for later use.	Supermarkets for ingredients.
Metamucil (Psyllium)	Procter & Gamble	Contains psyllium husk, a natural dietary fiber that relieves constipation and can lower blood cholesterol levels. Powder, granules, and wafer.	Pharmacies. Supermarkets. Online drugstores.
Miralax	Schering-Plough Healthcare Products	Used to relieve constipation with no harsh side effects. Powder laxative. Mixed with a liquid and taken by mouth one daily. Has no taste.	Pharmacies. Supermarkets. Online drugstores. 800-222-7579
Senakot	Purdue Pharma L.P.	Works by irritating bowel tissues resulting in bowel movements. Stimulant laxative. Tablet.	Pharmacies. Supermarkets. Online drugstores. 800-877-5666

Product	Source	Description	How to Access
Smooth Move herbal stimulant laxative tea	Traditional Medicinals Survivor input	Provides gentle and effective overnight relief. A sweet-tasting citrus-flavored herbal tea. Chocolate flavor also available.	Supermarkets. Whole Foods. Trader Joe's. Vitamin World. http://www.traditional medicinals.com http://www.drugstore.com

Products to Help Relieve Diarrhea

Product	Source	Description	How to Access
Imodium AD (loperamide)	McNeil Consumer Healthcare	Used to control diarrhea. Tablet, capsule, and liquid to take by mouth.	Pharmacies. Supermarkets. Online stores. 800-962-5357
Kaopectate	Chattem Inc.	Used to treat mild to moderate diarrhea. Chewable tablet, liquid. Take by mouth.	Pharmacies. Supermarkets. Online stores.
Lomotil (diphenoxylate with atropine)	Pfizer	Used to control diarrhea. Works by slowing the movement of the intestines. Tablet and liquid forms.	**Consult your physician. By prescription only.** 800-438-1985
Sandostatin (octreotide)	Novartis Pharmaceuticals	Helps control diarrhea and other symptoms of abdominal illness. Injection	**Consult your physician. By prescription only.**

Additional Side Effects of Treatment

Ear Pain and Hearing Loss

Description	How to Access
Radiation may cause swelling and obstruction of the eustachian tubes causing fluid to collect in the middle ear and/or swelling of the external ear canal. Usually temporary condition. Ventilation tubes may be necessary to relieve negative pressure when condition persists.	Consult your physician.
Fluid in the ear following head and neck surgery may occur following surgery on the maxillary sinus and palate. Usually a temporary condition. Ventilation tubes may be necessary to relieve negative pressure when condition persists.	Consult your physician.
Ear pain may be caused by hardening of the wax in the ear.	Consult your physician.
Ear pain may be caused by persistent tumor of the throat.	Consult your physician.
DermOtic Oil Fluocinolone acetonide oil 0.01% (ear drops)	Consult your physician

Loss of Smell and Taste

Description	How to Access
Loss of taste may occur as a result of mucositis and radiation effects on the taste buds (papillae). As papillae regenerate, sense of taste may return, usually after a few months.	Consult your radiation oncologist.
Loss of smell may be, in part, due to the loss of taste. Usually returns upon return of taste.	Consult your radiation oncologist.

Dry Eyes

Description	How to Access
Dry eyes may result from irradiation of the lacrimal (tear-producing) glands, which are located in the upper outer part of the eye sockets. They may be affected during treatment for cancers close to or involving the eyes or sinuses. Use of tear substitutes should be used to prevent dry eyes and further complications.	**Consult your ophthalmologist.**

Treating Toxicities From Targeted Therapies

Products to Help Treat Skin Rash

(Skin rash is a common side effect of treatment using targeted therapies.)

Product	Source	Description	How to Access
Aclovate (alclometasone dipropionate)	Nycomed USA	Used to treat skin problems that are accompanied by itching, redness, and swelling Synthetic corticosteroid. Cream, ointment.	**Consult your physician. By prescription only.** 800-645-9833
Atarax (hydroxyzine)	Pfizer	Use to relieve severe itching. Also used to relieve anxiety and tension. Has sedative effect.	**Consult your physician. By prescription only.** 800-438-1985

continues

Products to Help Treat Skin Rash *continued*

Product	Source	Description	How to Access
Bactroban Ointment (mupirocin)	GlaxoSmithKline (GSK)	Used to treat impetigo as well as other skin infections caused by bacteria. Ointment or cream	**Consult your physician. By prescription only.** 888-825-5249
Cipro (ciprofloxacin)	Bayer Pharmaceuticals	Used to treat infections caused by bacteria. An antibiotic. Tablet and suspension.	**Consult your physician. By prescription only.** 888-842-2937
Doryx (doxycxcyline)	Warner Chilcott Laboratories	Prevents the growth and spread of bacteria. Antibiotic taken by mouth to reduce inflammations of the skin. Pill or liquid form.	**Consult your physician. By prescription only.** (973) 442-3200
Dynacin (minocycline)	Medicis Pharmaceuticals Corp.	Used to treat bacterial infections, acne, and infections of the skin. A tetracycline antibiotic.	**Consult your physician. By prescription only.** 602-808-8800
Elidel (pimecrolimus 1% cream)	Novartis Pharmaceuticals	Shown to control the redness, inflammation, and itching of eczema. A topical cream.	**Consult your physician. By prescription only.** 800-277-2254
Metrogel (metronidazole gel, topical)	Galderma Laboratories LP	Used in the topical treatment of inflammatory lesions of the skin.	**Consult your physician. By prescription only.** 866-735-4137

Product	Source	Description	How to Access
Regenecare Wound Gel	MPM Medical Inc.	Used to reduce rash and itching caused by EGFR drugs. A pain-relieving hydrogel. Contains lidocaine HCl, collagen, and aloe vera.	**Consult your physician. By prescription only.** 800-232-5512 http://www.mpmmedical inc.com
Regenecare HA Wound Gel	MPM Medical Inc.	Used to treat skin problems such as itching and rash associated with EGFR drugs. Contains lidocaine HCl, collagen, aloe vera, and hyaluronic acid (HA).	**Consult your physician. By prescription only.** 800-232-5512. http://www.mpmmedical inc.com
Sumycin (tetracycline)	Par Pharmaceuticals Inc.	Used to reduce inflammations of the skin. Prevents growth and spread of bacteria. An antibiotic. Capsule and liquid.	**Consult your physician. By prescription only.** 800-828-9393
Terramycin (tetracycline)	Pfizer	Prevents the growth and spread of bacteria. Antibiotic taken by mouth to reduce inflammations of the skin. Pill or liquid form.	**Consult your physician. By prescription only.** 800-438-1985

283

Products to Help Relieve Itchy Dry Skin and Dry Nails

Product	Source	Description	How to Access
Aveeno Soothing Bath Treatment	Johnson & Johnson	Used for temporary relief of itchy, dry, sensitive skin. Fragrance-free with colloidal oatmeal.	Pharmacies. Supermarkets. Online drug stores.
Allegra	Sanofi-Aventis	Used for relief of dry itchy skin. An Antihistamine. May cause dry mouth. May cause drowsiness..	**Consult your physician. By prescription only.**
Baking soda baths	Survivor input	1 to 2 cups baking soda in lukewarm bath water. May help to reduce itchy skin.	Supermarkets for ingredients.
Benadryl	McNeil Consumer Healthcare	Used for relief of dry itchy skin. An Antihistamine. May cause dry mouth. May cause drowsiness.	Pharmacies. Supermarkets. Online drug stores. 888-222-6036
Carmol10	Doak Dermatologics	Used to help restore and retain normal skin softness. Total body lotion for dry skin. 10% urea.	Pharmacies. Online drug stores 800-405-3625
Claritin	Schering-Plough Health Care Products	Used for relief of dry, itchy skin. May cause dry mouth and drowsiness.	Pharmacies. Supermarkets. Online drug stores 800-222-7579

Product	Source	Description	How to Access
Clobex (clobetasol)	Galderma Laboratories, L.P.	Used for treatment of itchy, redness, dryness, crusting, scaling, inflammation, and discomfort of skin and scalp conditions. May also help relieve inflammation of nail areas. Cream or ointment.	**Consult your physician. By prescription only.** 866-735-4137
Dermovate (clobetasol)	Glaxo Smith Kline GSK	Used to treat itchy, redness, dryness, crusting, scaling, inflammation, and discomfort of skin and scalp conditions. May also help to relieve inflammation of nail areas. Cream or ointment.	**Consult your physician. By prescription only.** 888-825-5249
Dermablend concealment makeup	Dermablend	Does not contain fragrance or alcohol. Dermatologist tested, Allergy tested, Will not clog pores. Will not cause acne.	Online stores 800-662-8011 http://www.dermablend.com
Kenalog (triamcinolone)	Bristol-Myers Squibb Company	Used to treat the itching, redness, dryness, crusting, scaling, inflammation, and discomfort of various skin conditions. Helps reduce skin infections around the nails. A synthetic corticosteroid.	**Consult your physician. By prescription only.** 800-332-2056
Vanos (fluocinonide)	Medicis Pharmaceuticals Corp.	Used to treat the itching, redness, dryness, crusting, scaling, inflammation, and discomfort of various skin conditions. A synthetic corticosteroid cream.	**Consult your physician. By prescription only.** 800-550-5115

continues

Products to Help Relieve Itchy Dry Skin and Dry Nails *continued*

Product	Source	Description	How to Access
Lindi Face Serum	Lindi Skin Products	Used to hydrate the face, neck, shoulders, and upper body	800-380-4704 http://www.lindiskin.com Use online store locator.
Lindi Face Wash	Lindi Skin Products	Used to moisturize irritated and sensitive skin. Good for those with sensitivity to soap.	800-380-4704 http://www.lindiskin.com Use online store locator.
Lindi Lip Balm	Lindi Skin Products	Used to help with dry or cracked lips. May also help hydrate nail beds and cuticles.	800-380-4704 http://www.lindiskin.com Use online store locator.
Loprox (ciclopirox)	Medicis Pharmaceuticals Corp.	Used in the treatment of fungal and yeast infections of the skin. Topical cream, gel, or lotion.	**Consult your physician.** **By prescription only.**
Lyrica (Pregabalin)	Pfizer	Helps to control severe symptoms of itching.	**Consult your physician.** **By prescription only.** 800-438-1985
New-Skin Antiseptic Liquid Bandage	Medtech Labs Inc.	Apply to nail areas at first sign of skin cracking to prevent inflammation. Keeps out moisture, allowing the skin to heal.	Pharmacies. Supermarkets. Online drugstores.

Product	Source	Description	How to Access
Sarna Ultra Anti-Itch Cream	Stiefel Laboratories Inc.	Used to relieve itching associated with dry, rough, cracked skin.	Pharmacies. Online drugstores. 888-784-3335
Temovate (clobetasol propionate cream)	PharmaDerm	Used to treat itchiness, redness, dryness, crusting, scaling, inflammation, discomfort of various skin and scalp conditions. A synthetic corticosteroid. May also help to relieve inflammation of nail areas.	**Consult your physician.** **By prescription only.** 800-645-9833
Vinegar soaks	Home remedy	Helps to decrease nail disease and lowers risk of infection and spread of bacteria. Mix 1 part white vinegar with 10 parts water. Soak affected fingers or toes several times a day for 5 minutes or more.	Supermarket for ingredients.
Vistaril (hydroxyzine)	Pfizer	Used to relieve itchy skin. An antihistamine. Capsules 20 mg, 50 mg	**Consult your physician.** **By prescription only.** 800-438-1985
Westcort (hydrocortisone valerate steroid cream)	Ranbaxy USA Laboratories	Helps to relieve itching redness and swelling caused by a wide variety of skin conditions, such as acne-like rash. A synthetic (manmade) corticosteroid.	**Consult your physician.** **Prescription only.** 888-726-2299

Products to Help Moisturize and Heal Dry Skin and Nails

Product	Source	Description	How to Access
Aquaphor Healing Ointment	Eucerin	Protects dry, cracked or irritated skin to help enhance the natural healing process and restore smooth, healthy skin	Pharmacies. Supermarkets. Online drugstores. 800-227-4703 http://www.eucerinus.com
Aveeno Moisturizing Bar	Johnson & Johnson Consumer Products Companies	Moisturizes and cleanses dry, sensitive skin. Soap-free, hypoallergenic, formulated with natural oatmeal.	Pharmacies. Supermarkets. Online drugstores. 800-526-3967
Basis Sensitive Skin Bar Soap	Beiersdorf	Cleans dry, sensitive skin with almond oil, chamomile, and aloe vera.	Pharmacies. Supermarkets. Online drugstores. http://www.beiersdorf.com
Cetaphil Antibacterial Gentle Cleansing Bar	Galderma Laboratories, L.P	May be used to treat inflamed areas of the skin surrounding nails. Antibacterial soap for dry, sensitive skin.	Pharmacies. Supermarkets. Online drugstores. 866-735-4137
Cetaphil Gentle Cleansing Bar	Galderma Laboratories, L.P	Helps restore moisture and is a gentle, nonalkaline, nonsoap cleanser for dry, sensitive skin.	Pharmacies. Supermarkets. Online drugstores. 866-735-4137

Product	Source	Description	How to Access
Cetaphil Moisturizing Lotion	Galderma Laboratories, L.P	Helps restore skin's natural protective barrier. Fragrance free, non-comedogenic, non-greasy. moisturize skin and reduce itch.	Pharmacies. Supermarkets. Online drugstores. 866-735-4137
Cetaphil RESTORADEM	Galderma Laboratories, L.P	Skin Restoring Moisturizer with patented Filaggrin technology and ceramide technology is formulated to hydrate and soothe very dry, eczema-prone skin.	Pharmacies Online drugstores. 866-735-4137
Desenex	Novartis Consumer Health	Used in the treatment of superficial fungal infections of the skin. Relieves itching, burning and irritation. Antibiotic, anti-fungal powder, cream, spray.	Pharmacies. Supermarkets. Online drugstores. 800-277-2254
Dove Sensitive Skin Unscented Beauty Bar	Unilever	Moisturizes dry and sensitive skin. Helps to reduce itch. Fragrance-free hypoallergenic.	Pharmacies. Supermarkets. Online drugstores.
Eucerin Original	Eucerin	Heals and protects very dry sensitive skin. Fragrance-free, non-comedogenic, non-irritating. Lotion and Cream	Pharmacies. Supermarkets. Online drugstores. 800-227-4703 http://www.eucerinus.com

continues

Products to Help Moisturize and Heal Dry Skin and Nails *continued*

Product	Source	Description	How to Access
Lotrimin (clotrimozole)	Merck Consumer Health Products	Used to prevent nail areas from becoming infected. Antifungal ointment, cream, spray, powder.	Pharmacies. Supermarkets. Online drugstores. 800-898-8326
Neutrogena Facial Cleansing Bar	Neutrogena Corp.	Glycerine-rich bar that contains no harsh detergents, dyes, or hardeners. Dry skin, fragrance-free formula available.	Pharmacies. Supermarkets. Online drugstores. 800-582-4048
Neutrogena Norwegian Formula Hand Cream	Neutrogena Corp.	Helps heal dry, chapped hands. Concentrated, glycerine-rich formula.	Pharmacies. Supermarkets. Online drugstores. 800-582-4048
Neutrogena Ultra SheerDry-Touch Sunblock SPF 55 with Helioplex	Neutrogena Corp.	Offers protection for sensitive skin. Broad-spectrum UVA/UVB. PABA free. Helioplex helps prevent damaging UVA rays from penetrating deep under the skin's surface.	Pharmacies. Supermarkets Online drugstores. 800-582-4048
Vanicream Cleansing Bar	Pharmaceutical Specialties Inc.	Moisturizes while gently cleansing skin. Free of fragrance and common chemical irritants.	Pharmacies. 800-325-8232 http://www.psico.com

Product	Source	Description	How to Access
Vanicream Lite Lotion	Pharmaceutical Specialties Inc.	Moisturizes and soothes red, dry, irritated, cracking, or itchy skin.	Pharmacies. 800-325-8232 http://www.psico.com
Vanicream moisturizing skin cream	Pharmaceutical Specialties Inc.	Moisturizes and soothes red, irritated, cracking, or itchy skin.	Pharmacies. 800-325-8232 http://www.psico.com
Vanicream Sunscreen	Pharmaceutical Specialties Inc.	Protects skin from the sun without the use of sensitizing chemical sunscreens. Effectively blocks both UVA and UVB. Free of preservatives, dyes, perfume, lanolin, formaldehyde, PABA and benzophenones. 30, 35 and 60 SPF.	Pharmacies. 800-325-8232 http://www.psico.com
Vaseline Intensive Care Advanced Healing Lotion	Unilever	Hydrates and heals extra dry skin. Leaves skin feeling silky smooth and comfortable. Fragrance free.	Pharmacies. Supermarkets. Online drugstores. http://www.unilever.com
Vaseline Petroleum Jelly	Unilever	Apply a thick coat of Vaseline to hands and feet at night; cover with white cotton gloves and socks. Helps to moisturize and keep nails and skin from drying out.	Pharmacies. Supermarkets. Online drugstores. http://www.unilever.com

Alternative/Complementary Treatments That Survivors Have Found Helpful

Product	Source	Description	How to Access
Chinese herbal medicine	Survivor input	Refers to herbs used in combinations for many conditions. May be used to reduce pain, stiffness, fatigue, and inflammation.	**Consult your physician.** http://www.nccam.nih.gov
Chocolate	Survivor input	Mood soother	**Consult your physician.** Supermarkets. Convenience stores
Coffee	Survivor input	Mood soother	**Consult your physician.** Supermarkets. Convenience stores
Marshmallow Root Supplement	Survivor input	Considered a soothing and effective respiratory system supplement. As such, it aids the body in expelling excess fluid and mucus and will soothe the mucous membranes and a dry, hacking cough.	**Consult your physician.** Online stores http://www.herbal extractsplus
Massage	Survivor input	Refers to an assortment of techniques involving manipulation of the soft tissues of the body through pressure and movement.	**Consult your physician.** http://www.nccam.nih.gov

Product	Source	Description	How to Access
Meditation	Survivor input	Refers to a group of meditation techniques used for various health problems, including anxiety, pain depression, mood and self-esteem problems, stress, insomnia, and physical or emotional symptoms that may be associated with chronic illnesses and their treatment.	**Consult your physician.** http://www.nccam.nih.gov
Qigong	Survivor input	Refers to an energy modality involving the coordination of different breathing patterns with various physical postures and motions of the body to help improve health through the reduction of stress and exercise.	**Consult your physician.** http://www.nccam.nih.gov
Reflexology	Survivor input	Refers to a method of foot and hand massage in which pressure is applied to "reflex" zones of the feet and hands to help improve general health.	**Consult your physician.** http://www.nccam.nih.gov
Reiki	Survivor input	Refers to a healing energy that is channeled through a practitioner's hands. May induce relaxation; improve immunity; and reduce pain, stress, anxiety, and depression.	**Consult your physician.** http://www.nccam.nih.gov

continues

Alternative/Complementary Treatments That Survivors Have Found Helpful *continued*

Product	Source	Description	How to Access
Tai chi	Survivor input	Refers to moving the body slowly and gently, while breathing deeply and meditating. Used to improve physical condition, muscle strength, coordination, and flexibility. Also used to ease pain and stiffness.	**Consult your physician.** http://www.nccam.nih.gov
Tea with Honey and Cream	Survivor input	May help to heal mouth sores. Also helps mood and well-being	**Consult your physician.** Supermarkets Convenience stores
Yoga	Survivor input	Refers to a mind-body medicine typically focusing on intervention strategies that are thought to promote health and well-being.	**Consult your physician.** http://www.nccam.nih.gov

Miscellaneous

Product	Source	Description	How to Access
Disposable Bed Pads Underpads	Multiple manufacturers Survivor input	Can be placed on pillow while sleeping to keep pillow dry. Can be used while under-going radiation treatment and coughing at night. Large rectangular pad normally used on beds for bed-bound patients.	Pharmacies. Online stores.
Headwrap or JawBra with Gel Packs	CranioMandibular Rehab, Inc.	Helps decrease swelling and pain in face and jaw after surgery or radiation with soft hot/cold gel packs and compression.	**Consult your physician.** 800-206-8381 http://www.Craniorehab.com
Humidifier	Many brands Survivor input	Helps to improve air quality and adds moisture to bedroom assisting sleeping patient with xeroxtomia (dry mouth)	Pharmacies. Department Stores. Online stores.
Industrial Strength Blender	Multiple manufacturers Survivor input	Used to puree foods for people who have swallowing difficulties. Has more power than a commercial blender.	Online stores.
Kat Von D Tattoo Concealer	Sephora Survivor input	Formulated to cover tattoos, can also be used to cover scars.	Sephora Stores 877-737-4672 http://www.SEPHORA.com
Universal Facial Wrap	ClearPoint Medical Survivor input	Elastic bandage can be wrapped around face/neck while sleeping to reduce swelling.	Plastic surgeon's office 866-694-7799 http://www.clearpointmd.com

Appendix

PROGRAMS OF OUTREACH AND SUPPORT, LITERATURE, WEB SITES, AND ORGANIZATIONS

Support for People with Oral and Head and Neck Cancer (SPOHNC), a patient-directed self-help organization, was founded in 1991 by an oral cancer survivor. This nonprofit organization is dedicated to raising awareness and meeting the emotional, physical, and humanistic needs of oral and head and neck cancer patients, their families and friends.

SPOHNC offers two programs of outreach and support for patients with oral and head and neck cancer. Its National Survivor Volunteer Network (NSVN) is a network of more than 125 survivor volunteers who communicate on a one-to-one basis with newly diagnosed patients and recovering survivors. Patients may phone 1-800-377-0928 or e-mail info@spohnc.org to be matched with a volunteer who can provide information, support, and encouragement to those in need.

Chapters of SPOHNC are found throughout the United States. These chapters hold monthly meetings offering information, support, and encouragement to newly diagnosed patients, survivors, family members, and friends in a friendly and non-threatening forum. Survivors share their situations, experiences, coping strategies, and hopes. Educational presentations by health care professionals are also part of the SPOHNC program. Some chapters are facilitated by health care professionals, and others are facilitated by cancer survivors. SPOHNC chapters strive to provide survivors a support system tailored to their individual needs.

Following is a list of SPOHNC chapters. In some cities, there is more than one chapter. A complete listing of chapters and contact information can be found on SPOHNC's Web site at http://www.spohnc.org. Additional information about specific chapters can also be obtained by calling SPOHNC's office at 1-800-377-0928.

Arizona—Chandler

Arizona—Phoenix/Mesa

Arizona- Phoenix

Arizona—Scottsdale

Arkansas—Northwest

California—Los Angeles

California—Orange County

California—Paso Robles

California—San Diego

California- Santa Maria

California—Stanford

California—Ventura

Colorado—Denver

Connecticut—New Haven

Connecticut—New London

Connecticut—Norwich

DC—Georgetown

DC—Washington

Florida—Boca Raton

Florida—Englewood

Florida- Fort Myers

Florida—Fort Walton Beach

Florida—Gainesville

Florida—Lecanto

Florida—Miami

Florida—Naples

Florida—Ocala

Florida—Sarasota

Florida—Wellington

Georgia—Atlanta

Georgia—Atlanta/Emory

Georgia—Augusta

Georgia—Columbus

Illinois—Chicago

Illinois—Evanston/Highland Park

Illinois—Maywood

Indiana—Fort Wayne

Indiana—Indy/North

Indiana—Terre Haute

Iowa—Des Moines

Kansas—Kansas City

Louisiana—Baton Rouge

Maine—Augusta

Maryland—Baltimore

Massachusetts—Boston

Massachusetts—Cape Cod

Massachusetts—Danvers

Michigan—Detroit

Michigan—St. Joseph

Michigan—Troy

Minnesota—Minneapolis

Missouri—St. Louis

Montana—Bozeman

Nebraska—Omaha

New Jersey—Long Branch

New Jersey—Morristown

New Jersey—Princeton

New Jersey—Sommerville

New Jersey—Toms River

New Mexico—Albuquerque

New York—Albany

New York—Buffalo

New York—Manhattan

New York—New Hyde Park

New York—Rochester

New York—Stony Brook

New York—Syosset

New York—Westchester

North Carolina- Ashville

North Carolina—Chapel Hill/ Durham

North Carolina—Charlotte

Ohio—Cincinnati

Ohio—Cleveland

Ohio—Dayton

Ohio—Lima

Oklahoma—Tulsa

Oregon—Medford

Oregon—The Williamette Valley

Pennsylvania—Harrisburg

Pennsylvania—Monroeville

Pennsylvania—New Castle

Pennsylvania—Philadelphia

Pennsylvania—York

Tennessee—Chattanooga

Tennessee—Nashville

Texas—Dallas

Texas—Fort Worth

Texas—Houston/Tomball

Texas—McAllen

Texas—Plano

Virginia—Charlottesville

Virginia—Fairfax

Virginia—Norfolk

Washington—Seattle

Wisconsin—Madison

Wisconsin—Milwaukee

Autobiographies of Head and Neck Survivors

Achatz, G., & Kokonas, N. (2011). *Life, on the line, a chef's story of chasing greatness, facing death and redefining the way we eat.* New York, NY: Penguin Group, Inc.

Brook, I. (2009). *My voice: A physician's personal experience with throat cancer.* Seattle, WA. Available at http://www.createspace.com, or E-read at http://dribrook.blogspot.com.

Cohn, H. (2006). *Risen from the ashes—Tales of a musical messenger.* Lanham, MD: Hamilton Books.

Fleming, T. (1999). *A rendezvous with clouds.* Albuquerque, NM: University of New Mexico Press.

Healey, T. (2006). *At face value—My triumph over a disfiguring cancer.* Ashland, OR: Caveat Press.

Hess, P. (2003). *The battle is won because of who God is.* Richardson, TX: Angel Hearts Publishing.

Hess, P. (2011). *It's all about God (Addendum).* Richardson, TX: Angel Hearts Publishing.

Hinz, D. (2011). *My private mountain.* Philadelphia, PA: Dorrance Publishing. E-read http://www.davehinzfoundation.com.

Phelan, W. A. (2006). *Running with cancer: The ultimate marathon.* Bloomington, IN: AuthorHouse.

Books and DVDs About
Oral and Head and Neck Cancer

American Cancer Society (n.d.). *Atlas of clinical oncology* [Series]. Hamilton, Ontario, Canada: B. C. Decker.

Clarke, L. K., & Dropkin, M. J. (2006). *Head and neck cancer.* Pittsburgh, PA: Oncology Nursing Society.

Clifford Chao, K. S., & Ozyigit, G. (Eds.). (2003). *Intensity modulated radiation therapy.* Philadelphia, PA: Lippincott Williams & Wilkins.

Harrison, L. B., Sessions, R. B., & Hong, W. K. (2004). *Head and neck cancer, a multidisciplinary approach.* Philadelphia, PA: Lippincott Williams & Wilkins.

Leupold, N. E. (Ed.). (2006). *Eat well—Stay nourished, a recipe and resource guide for coping with eating challenges.* Lenexa, KS: Cookbook Publishers.

Leupold, N. E., & Sciubba, J. J. (Eds.). (2008). *Meeting the challenges of oral and head and neck cancer: A survivor's guide.* San Diego, CA: Plural Publishing.

Leupold, N. E., & Sciubba, J. J. (Eds.). (2011). *Meeting the challenges of oral and head and neck cancer: A guide for survivors and caregivers.* San Diego, CA: Plural Publishing.

Lydiatt, W., & Johnson, P. (2001). *Cancers of the mouth and throat, a patient's guide.* Omaha, NE: Addicus Books.

Shah, J. P. (Ed.). (2001). *Cancer of the head and neck,* a volume in the American Cancer Society *Atlas of Clinical Oncology* series. Hamilton, Ontario, Canada: BC Decker.

Support for People with Head Neck Cancer (SPOHNC) & Bristol Myers Squibb. (2006). *We have walked in your shoes.* Locust Valley, NY: Author.

St. Mary's Regional Cancer Center. (2011). *Head and neck cancer education* DVD. Grand Junction, CO. Call 1-970-298-2351 or e-mail Debra.Hesse@stmarygj.org to request copies.

THANC. (2007). *Words to Live By–Patients helping patients on their journey with head and neck cancer.* DVD. New York, NY: Call 1-212-844-6832 or e-mail info@thancfoundation.org to request copies.

THANC. (2007). *Words to Live By–Patients helping patients on their journey with thyroid cancer.* DVD. New York, NY: Call 1-212-844-6832 or e-mail info@thancfoundation.org to request copies.

Wang, C. (1996). *Radiation therapy for head and neck neoplasms.* New York, NY: Wiley-Liss.

Books and Magazines About Cancer

Anderson, G., & Simonton, C. (1999). *Cancer: 50 essential things to do.* New York, NY: Plume.

Armstrong, L. (2001). *It's not about the bike: My journey back to life.* New York, NY: Berkley Trade.

Aron, L. (2010). *Your write to heal.* Raleigh, NC: Lulu Publishing. Available at http://www.writerwithinworkshops.com

Canfield, J. (1996). *Chicken soup for the soul: 101 healing stories about those who have survived cancer.* Deerfield, FL: HCI.

Coping with Cancer magazine, P.O. Box 682268, Franklin, TN 37068-2268; 615-790-2400; http://www.coping.com

CURE magazine, 33201 Oak Lawn Avenue Suite 610, Dallas, TX 75219; 800-210-CURE; http://www.curetoday.com

DeSimone, D. (2011). *From stage IV to center stage.* Carlsbad, CA: Balboa Press—A division of Hay House Publishers.

Fincannon, J. L., & Bruss, K. V. (2003). *Couples confronting cancer: Keeping your relationship strong.* Atlanta, GA: American Cancer Society.

Geffen, J. (2000). *The journey through cancer.* New York, NY: Crown.

Granet, R. (2001). *Surviving cancer emotionally: Learning how to heal.* New York, NY: John Wiley & Sons.

Grayzel, E. (2010) *You are not alone: Families touched by cancer.* Ashland, OH: Atlas.

Groopman, J. (2004). *The anatomy of hope.* New York, NY: Random House.

Heal—Living Well After Cancer magazine, 3500 Maple Avenue, Suite 750, Dallas, TX 75219; 800-210-2873; http://www.healtoday.com

Hermann, J. F. (2001). *Cancer in the family: Helping children cope with a parent's illness.* Atlanta, GA: American Cancer Society.

Hoffman, B. (1996). *A cancer survivor's almanac: Charting your journey.* Minneapolis, MN: Chronimed.

Holland, J. C., & Lewis, S. (2001). *The human side of cancer: Living with hope, coping with uncertainty.* New York, NY: Harper.

Kabat-Zinn, J. (1990). *Full catastrophe living: Using the wisdom of your body and mind to face pain, stress and illness.* New York, NY: Bantam Dell.

Kushner, H. S. (2004). *When bad things happen to good people.* New York, NY: Anchor.

Schlessel Harpham, W. (1997). *When a parent has cancer: A guide to caring for your children.* New York, NY; Harper Collins.

Schlessel Harpham, W. (2003). *Diagnosis: Cancer* (exp. ed.). New York, NY: W.W. Norton.

Schlessel Harpham, W. (2005). *Happiness in a storm.* New York, NY: W.W. Norton.

Treadway, D. (2010). *Home before dark: A family portrait of cancer and healing.* New York, NY: Union Square Press.

Zakarian, B. (1996). *Activist cancer patient: How to take charge of your treatment.* New York, NY: John Wiley & Sons.

Organizations for Oral and Head and Neck Cancer Information

Adenoid Cystic Carcinoma Organization International (ACCOI)
PO Box 112186
Tacoma, WA 98411
1-888-223-7983
http://www.accoi.org

Adenoid Cystic Carcinoma Research Foundation (ACCRF)
PO Box 442
Needham, MA 02494
781-248-9699
http://www.accrf.org

American Academy of Otolaryngology-Head and Neck Surgery (AAO-HNS)
1650 Diagonal Road
Alexandria, VA 22314-2857
703-836-4444
http://www.entnet.org

American Association for Cancer Research (AACR)
615 Chestnut Street, 17th Floor
Philadelphia, PA 19106
215-440-9300/866-423-3695
http://www.aacr.org

American Cancer Society (ACS)
250 Williams Street NW
Atlanta, GA 30303-1002
800-227-2345
http://www.cancer.org

American Head & Neck Society (AHNS)
11300 W. Olympic Boulevard, Suite 600
Los Angeles, CA 90064
310-437-0559
http://www.ahns.info

American Institute for Cancer Research (AICR)
1759 R Street, NW

Washington, DC 20009
800-843-8114
http://www.aicr.org

American Society of Clinical Oncology (ASCO)
2318 Mill Rd. Suite 800
Alexandria, VA 22314
888-282-2552
http://www.asco.org

American Society for Therapeutic Radiology & Oncology (ASTRO)
8280 Willow Oaks Corporate Drive, Suite 500
Fairfax, VA 22031
800-962-7876
703-502-1550
http://www.astro.org

Cancer Care
275 Seventh Avenue
New York, NY 10001
800-813-HOPE (800-813-4673)
212-712-8400
http://www.cancercare.org

Cancer.net
2318 Mill Road
Suite 800
Alexandria, VA 22314
888-651-3038
http://www.cancer.net

CarePages
345 Hudson Street
16th Floor
New York, NY 10014
888-852-5521
http://www.carepages.com

Head & Neck Cancer Alliance
135 Rutledge Avenue MSC 550

Charleston, SC 29425-550
866-792-4622
http://www.headandneck.org

International Association of Laryngectomees (IAL)
925B Peachtree Street
NE Suite 316
Atlanta, GA 30309
866-425-3678
http://www.theial.com

National Cancer Institute (NCI)
Office of Communications & Education
Public Inquiries Office
6116 Executive Boulevard, Suite 300
Bethesda, MD 20892-8322
800-4-CANCER (800-422-6237)
http://www.cancer.gov

National Institute of Dental and Craniofacial Research (NIDCR)
Bethesda, MD 20892
301-496-4261
http://www.nidcr.nih.gov

Oral Cancer Foundation
3419 Via Lido #205
Newport Beach, CA 92663
949-646-8000
http://www.oralcancerfoundation.org

Society of Otorhinolaryngology and Head-Neck Nurses (SOHN)
207 Downing Street
New Smyrna Beach, FL 32168
386-428-1695
http://www.sohnnurse.com

Support for People with Oral and Head and Neck Cancer (SPOHNC)
P.O. Box 53, Locust Valley, NY 11560
800-377-0928
http://www.spohnc.org

WebWhispers
PO Box 9443
Longview TX 75608-9443
1-800-321-0591
http://www.webwhispers.org

Helpful Organizations

Air Care Alliance (ACA)
State Hwy 595
Lindrith, NM 87029
888-260-9707
http://www.aircareall.org

American Dental Association (ADA)
211 East Chicago Ave.
Chicago, IL 60611-2678
312-440-2500
http://www.ada.org

American Dietetic Association
120 South Riverside Plaza, Ste. 2000
Chicago, IL 60606-6995
800-877-1600
http://www.eatright.org

American Pain Foundation (APF)
201 N. Charles St., Ste. 710
Baltimore, MD 21201
888-615-7246
http://www.painfoundation.org

American Psychosocial Oncology Society (APOS)
154 Hansen Rd., Ste. 201
Charlottesville, VA 22911
1-866-276-7443
434-293-5350
http://www.apos-society.org

Association of Clinicians for the Underserved (ACU)
1420 Spring Hill Rd., Ste. 600
Tysons Corner, VA 22102
703-442-5318
http://www.clinicians.org

Association of Oncology Social Work (AOSW)
100 N. 20 St. Ste. 400
Philadelphia, PA 19103
215-599-6093
http://www.aosw.org

Cancer Fund of America (CFA)
2901 Breezewood Ln.
Knoxville, TN 37921
800-578-5284
http://www.cfoa.org

Cancer Legal Resource Center (CLRC)
919 Albany St.
Los Angeles, CA 90015
1-866-843-2572
http://www.CancerLegalResourceCenter.org

Cancer Patient Education Network (CPEN)
154 Hansen Rd., Ste. 201
Charlottesville, VA 22911
434-284-4697
http://www.cancerpatienteducation.org

Cancer Support Community (CSC)
1050 17 St. NW
Washington, DC 20036
888-793-9355
http://www.cancersupportcommunity.org

Catholic Charities USA (CCUSA)
66 Canal Center Plaza, Ste. 600
Alexandria, Virginia 22314
Phone: (703) 549-1390

Fax: (703) 549-1656
http://www.catholiccharitiesusa.org

Chronic Disease Fund (CDF)
6900 N. Dallas Pkwy., Ste. 200
Plano, TX 75024
877-968-7233
http://www.cdfund.org

Corporate Angel Network Inc. (CAN)
Westchester County Airport
One Loop Rd.
White Plains, NY 10604
866-328-1313
914-328-1313
http://www.corpangelnetwork.org

Education Network to Advance Cancer Clinical Trials (ENACCT)
7625 Wisconsin Ave., 3rd Floor
Bethesda, MD 20814
240-482-4730
http://www.enacct.org

Fertile Hope
2201 E. 6th St.
Austin, TX 78702
855-220-7777
http://www.livestrong.org/fertilehope

Gilda's Club Worldwide
48 Wall St., 11th Floor
New York, NY 10005
888-445-3248
917-305-1200
http://www.gildasclub.org

Healthwell Foundation
PO Box 4133
Gaithersburg, MD 20878
(800) 675-8416
http://www.healthwellfoundation.org

Intercultural Cancer Council (ICC)
1709 Dryden Rd. Ste. 1025
Houston, TX 77030
713-798-4614
http://www.iccnetwork.org

Joe's House
505 E. 79 St., Ste. 17E
NY, NY 10075
877-563-7468
http://www.joeshouse.org

Kids Konnected
26071 Merit Circle, Ste. 103
Laguna Hills, CA 92653
800-899-2866
http://www.kidskonnected.org

Lance Armstrong Foundation
2201 E. Sixth St.
Austin, TX 78702
877-236-8820
866-673-7205
http://www.livestrong.org

Look Good . . . Feel Better
c/o Personal Care Products Council Foundation
1101 17th Street NW, Ste. 300
Washington, DC 20036
800-395-5665
http://www.lookgoodfeelbetter.org

Lotsa Helping Hands
2 Clock Tower Place, Ste. 610
Maynard, MA 01754
http://www.lotsahelpinghands.com

My Lifeline.org Cancer Foundation
55 Madison St., Ste. 750
Denver, CO 80206

303-549-0405
http://www.mylifeline.org

MedlinePlus—Trusted Health Information for You
A Service of the U.S. National Library of Medicine and the
National Institutes of Health
8600 Rockville Pike
Bethesda, MD 20894
http://www.medlineplus.gov

National Association for Home Care (NAHC)
228 Seventh St., SE
Washington, DC 20003
202-547-7424
http://www.nahc.org

National Association of Social Workers (NASW)
750 First St., NE, Ste. 700
Washington, DC 20002-4241
800-638-8799
202-408-8600
http://www.naswdc.org

National Cancer Institute's Cancer Information Service (CIS)
6116 Executive Blvd., Ste. 300
Bethesda, MD 20892-8322
800-4-cancer (800-422-6237)
http://www.cancer.gov/aboutnci/cis

National Coalition for Cancer Survivorship (NCCS)
1010 Wayne Ave. Ste. 770
Silver Spring, MD 20910
888-650-9127
http://www.canceradvocacy.org

National Comprehensive Cancer Network (NCCN)
275 Commerce Dr.
Suite 300
Fort Washington, PA 19034
215-690-0300
http://www.nccn.org

National Family Caregivers Association (NFCA)
10400 Connecticut Ave., Ste. 500
Kensington, MD 20895-3944
800-896-3650
301-942-6430
http://www.nfcacares.org

National Library of Medicine (NLM)
8600 Rockville Pike
Bethesda, MD 20894
888-346-3656
301-594-5983
http://www.nlm.nih.gov

National Organization for Rare Disorders (NORD)
55 Kenosia Ave.
PO Box 1968
Danbury, CT 06813-1968
203-744-0100
http://www.rarediseases.org

NeedyMeds
PO Box 219
Gloucester, MA 01931
http://www.needymeds.com

The Oley Foundation
214 Hun Memorial, MC-28 Albany Medical Center
Albany, NY
1-800-776-6539
http://www.oley.org

Partnership for Prescription Assistance (PPA)
1100 15th St., NW
Washington, DC 20005
888-4PPA-NOW (477-2669)
http://www.pparx.org

Patient Access Network Foundation (PAN)
PO Box 221858
Charlotte, NC 28222

866-316-PANF (7263)
http://www.panfoundation.org

Patient Advocate Foundation (PAF)
421 Butler Farm Rd.
Hampton, VA 23666
800-532-5274
http://www.patientadvocate.org

Patient Power
9220 SE 68th St.
Mercer Island, WA 98040-5135
http://www.patientpower.info

Patient Resource
PO Box 860487
Shawnee, KS 66286
816-333-3595
http://www.patientresource.net

R.A. Bloch Cancer Foundation
One H & R Block Way
Kansas City, MO 64105
800-433-0464
816-854-5050
http://www.blochcancer.org

RadiologyInfo
820 Jorie Blvd.
Oak Brook, IL 60523
630-571-2670
http://www.radiologyinfo.org

Research Advocacy Network
6505 W. Park Blvd., Ste. 305
Plano, TX 75093
877-276-2187
http://www.researchadvocacy.org

Strength for Life
902 Constance Lane

Port Jefferson Station, NY 11776
631-675-6513
http://www.strengthforlifeny.org

Surveillance Epidemiology and End Results (SEER)
National Cancer Institute
Suite 504, MSC 8316
6116 Executive Boulevard
Bethesda, MD 20892-8316
301-496-8510
http://www.seer.cancer.gov

The LGBT Cancer Project
136 W. 16th St. 1E
NY, NY 10011
212-675-2633
http://www.lgbtcancer.org

The Wellness Community
1050 17th St. NW
Washington, DC 20036
888-793-WELL (888-793-9355)
202-659-9709
http://www.thewellnesscommunity.org

US Department of Veteran Affairs (VA)
810 Vermont Ave. NW
Washington, DC 20420
800-827-1000
http://www.va.gov

US Oncology
10101 Woodloch Forest
The Woodlands, TX 77380
800-381-2637
http://www.usoncology.com

Vital Options International & The Group Room
4419 Coldwater Canyon Ave., Ste. I
Studio City, CA 91604
800-477-7666
http://www.vitaloptions.org

INDEX